A Multidisciplinary Approach
to Health Care Ethics

A Multidisciplinary Approach to Health Care Ethics

Drew E. Hinderer
Saginaw Valley State University, Michigan

Sara R. Hinderer
Saint Mary's of Saginaw, Michigan

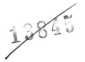

Mayfield Publishing Company
Mountain View, California
London • Toronto

Library of Congress Cataloging-in-Publication Data
Hinderer, Drew E.
   A multidisciplinary approach to health care ethics / Drew E. Hinderer, Sara R. Hinderer.
      p. cm.
   Includes index.
   ISBN 0-7674-1302-4
   1. Medical ethics. 2. Medical ethics—Case studies. I. Hinderer, Sara R. II. Title.

R724.H55 2000
174'.2—dc21   00-024568
                                                                                        CIP

Manufactured in the United States of America
10   9   8   7   6   5   4   3   2   1

Mayfield Publishing Company
1280 Villa Street
Mountain View, CA 94041

Sponsoring editor, Ken King; production editor, Deneen M. Sedlack; manuscript editor, Joan Pendleton; art and design manager, Jean Mailander; text and cover designer, Michael Warrell; manufacturing manager, Randy Hurst. The text was set in 10/12.5 Palatino by Shepherd, Inc. and printed on acid-free, 50# Finch Opaque by Malloy Lithographing, Inc.

CONTENTS

PART III
Health Care Issues for Discussion 111

CHAPTER TEN
Confidentiality, Patients, and Staff   169

PREFACE

There are so many excellent biomedical ethics books that offering a new text requires some explanation. As college teachers, and also as health care professionals, we came to feel that three important needs have largely gone unmet by existing texts, as good as they are in other respects. These needs concern the kinds of issues and cases covered, the practical application of course materials to contemporary health care practice, and the audience for texts in health care ethics. Briefly, we think too much time is often spent on high-profile issues that most health care practitioners will seldom, if ever, encounter, while not enough stress is placed on the sorts of clinical ethical issues that arise in everyday practice across the many health care disciplines. We also think that discussions and procedures that enable students to resolve ethical issues responsibly are more valuable for most health care students than are presentations of issues emphasizing the diversity of ethical analyses. And we think it is important to offer students in the first few years of college the opportunity to think carefully about ethical issues without presupposing advanced reading competence or a particular disciplinary affiliation. Accordingly, *A Multidisciplinary Approach to Health Care Ethics* addresses ethical issues in practice situations, in ways that sharpen analytical skills and responsible decision making, from a multidisciplinary perspective.

The world of health care is undergoing profound and dramatic changes. New technologies such as those associated with the Genome Project raise ethical puzzles; issues like physician-assisted suicide grab the headlines in sensational media coverage; and political struggles over patients' rights and managed care are fought to stalemate in legislatures around the nation. Health care professionals certainly need to be able to speak to those issues responsibly, and we address some of them in this text. But there are also many ethical issues of daily concern to health care professionals that are less visible to the general public: how to counsel the prospective parents of a child with probable genetic birth defects, whether to authorize a coronary bypass on the elderly Alzheimer's patient, and what to do about the home-care patient who might (or might not) be abused, for example. Should the stroke victim be allowed to return to his job as a truck driver? What should we do about the impaired colleague or the minor medication error that, if reported, will cost a friend her job? Why shouldn't the occupational therapist date her former client? Such issues may have a lower profile in the public consciousness, but they are the moment-to-moment ethical problems of professionals in practice. Health care professionals also need to be able to address these issues responsibly. So, in *A Multidisciplinary Approach* we present a balance of both kinds of issues, emphasizing cases likely to occur in normal practice.

Moreover, ethical issues need to be *resolved*, not just discussed. It is important to understand the diversity of responsible arguments on many sides of high-profile ethics and public policy issues and to develop and articulate well-considered positions on those issues. But it is also important to decide day-to-day ethical issues sensitively, responsibly, and effectively. Accordingly, we discuss the *practical* advantages and deficiencies of various ethical decision-making approaches as ways of resolving real problems, providing enough theoretical groundwork to avoid superficiality and evasion, but not so much as to lose beginning students. We also discuss relationships among ethics and law, religion, codes of ethics, "rights talk," and the practices of peers in light of the ways such matters intersect with efforts to resolve ethical problems in health care practice.

Virtually all health care practitioners deliver care within the context of complex institutions. Accrediting agencies, such as the Joint Commission for Accrediting Health Care Organizations, increasingly insist on effective, multidisciplinary mechanisms for addressing ethical issues. Moreover, we think it is absolutely essential for health care professionals across the disciplines to be able to work collaboratively to resolve problems. Accordingly, our approach to resolving ethical issues stresses multidisciplinary collaboration, both formally, in the work of institutional ethics committees, and informally.

Finally, we recognize that many students considering careers in health care will pursue two-year professional programs, while many more will need to devote all or most of their upper-level college course work to their disciplinary specialties. Accordingly, *A Multidisciplinary Approach* is written to be accessible to first- and second-year college students. It does not require, though it does encourage, familiarity with journal articles in the health care disciplines; nor does it presuppose a sophisticated vocabulary or background in a specific health care field. By drawing all cases from actual clinical experiences across the diverse fields of health care practice and presenting them in an accessible way, we hope students will recognize themselves as participants in ethical decision making regardless of their prospective career choices and levels of education.

A Multidisciplinary Approach to Health Care Ethics is structured in three parts. Chapters 1 through 3 address what ethical issues are; why they are often difficult to resolve; how they relate to legal, religious, and other matters; and how they can be resolved in a practical and ethically responsible way. Chapters 4 through 6 discuss ethical decision-making perspectives that are common but flawed, such as egoism and some forms of relativism, and perspectives that contribute usefully to the decision procedure offered in Chapter 3: a modified form of consequentialism, principled reasoning, and a combination of virtue ethics with feminism. Chapters 7 through 10 present four major health care issues and invite careful analysis and further research: access to health care and considerations of social justice; genetic research, especially that affecting reproductive choices; euthanasia and physician-assisted suicide; and privacy and confidentiality. Each chapter includes opportunities for extensive practice in ethical reasoning by means of cases and other issues for discussion.

The authors are profoundly indebted to our many friends and colleagues across the health care disciplines, even though we can mention only a few by name. We extend particular thanks to Gaye Freeman, M.D., who got us started in clinical ethics, as well as Leonard Fleck, Ph.D., and Howard Brody, M.D., at Michigan State University, and our colleagues at Saginaw Valley State University in the Crystal M. Lange College of Nursing and Allied Health Sciences, including, especially, Crystal Lange, R.N., herself. We are deeply grateful to Lori and Grant Crago, M.D.s, for several cases, and to Chris Chesny, R.N., and Judith Davidson, ACSW, for many more, as well as for modeling professionalism and ethical sensitivity.

All the cases in *A Multidisciplinary Approach to Health Care Ethics* are drawn from our clinical practice in eight hospitals, five universities, and several other settings. While readers may think they recognize colleagues (or even themselves) in these cases, we have been very cautious to conceal the identities of those involved: any resemblance of characters, places, and incidents in this book to any real person, location, or event is entirely coincidental.

PART I

Ethical Issues and Related Matters

In the following three chapters we begin to think about health care issues from a new perspective, one that we are calling *A Multidisciplinary Approach to Health Care Ethics*. In Chapter 1, we meet some common ethical issues and determine what makes them *ethical* problems. We also explore what to expect out of studying ethics and try our hands at resolving some ethical issues that occur in health care practice. In Chapter 2, we explore the relationship between health care ethics and other issues, such as role-based expectations, personal feelings, legal obligations, religious faith, people's rights, codes of ethics, and current standards of practice. In each case, we discover that while roles, feelings, laws, and the rest are important, none is a fully responsible substitute for multidisciplinary ethical reasoning. Accordingly, in Chapter 3, we present a more adequate model for ethical problem solving and apply it to two ethical problems. Our approach relies on six steps: problem identification, values identification, consequence identification, option selection, and documentation.

Throughout this book, we present many case studies for analysis and discussion. These case studies are real cases, in that each of them has come up (some of them repeatedly) in our practice of health care. However, details of most of these cases have been simplified, and events have been disguised to protect the confidentiality of those who actually participated in them. Sometimes, this may tempt you to wonder about information that was left out or to "poke holes" in the case studies. You will find them much more useful, however, if you focus on the ethical problem illustrated by the case studies and think about how such cases could happen, rather than worrying too much about details you might question.

Finally, we encourage you to "get into" this material. Many of the issues you will encounter in *A Multidisciplinary Approach to Health Care Ethics* are issues that you will run into repeatedly during your career.

1

You may find that you disagree with other students about some issues, and you may find that you disagree with some suggestions we make about what constitutes responsible ethical reasoning. You may even feel a little uncomfortable with some of this material. For better or worse, that is the nature of ethical issues: they can be uncomfortable and controversial. Remember that there can be more than one responsible way to resolve an ethical issue. The goal of this book is not to guarantee universal agreement, or to make sure everyone is comfortable, but to help students develop skillful, professionally responsible ethical reasoning.

CHAPTER ONE

Ethics: What, Why, and Why Now?

GETTING STARTED: INTRODUCTORY CASE STUDIES

Case 1.1: Conflict in Professional Responsibility

As the occupational therapist principally responsible for working with 55-year-old Mr. Slawinski, you have a deep sense of how important self-sufficiency is to his self-esteem and self-respect. He has made good progress in rehabilitation from a series of mild strokes, but continues to suffer occasional episodes of confusion, memory loss, coordinational deficiencies, and inattentiveness. He is, however, eager to resume his normal life and return to his job as a heavy-equipment operator; and he adamantly insists that he's well enough to drive a car. Should you approve his discharge and certify him to drive?

Case 1.2: Justice Versus Patients' Wishes

Jack Stone is the 17-year-old victim of a motorcycle accident and will probably not live more than about six hours, due to massive head injuries. As a strong advocate of organ donation, you are pleased that Jack's family has consented to allow the Midstate Organ Procurement Agency to retrieve skin, bone, marrow, and any undamaged organs for transplantation to patients on the regional waiting list. Under normal circumstances, these are allocated according to medical need and probability of success, length of time on the waiting list, and other criteria. But you have recently learned that a famous guitarist has entered your hospital and is in need of a liver transplant, his own liver having been destroyed by chronic alcoholism and drug abuse. Should the family be informed so that they can consider allocating Jack's organs to the rock star?

Case 1.3: Sanctity of Life Versus Economic Costs

Ms. Ashley has been in a persistent vegetative state since she was severely injured in an automobile accident. Kept alive by means of a comprehensive life-support system, she has only a minimal probability of any form of improvement. Ms. Ashley is uninsured, and her care is extremely expensive: about $1,100 a day, counting staff time as well as the costs associated with the machinery. Moreover, since the equipment used by Ms. Ashley is unavailable to any other patients, the hospital would probably not have enough life-support systems available should a number of patients arrive at once, as a result of a multi-car accident, for example. Ms. Ashley is now developing a serious bacterial infection that is potentially fatal if left untreated. Should it be treated?

Some Key Ideas and Definitions

Most reasonable people will find these three cases troubling. Each one involves an apparent conflict between differing values; each also appears to require making a choice between those differing values that involves sacrificing at least some values. In other words, each involves an ethical dilemma.

> Here are two key ideas in this section. A conflict in values is a situation where human interests and concerns cannot all be accommodated. An ethical dilemma is a conflict among values that poses a problem in making decisions based on standards of fairness, justice, rightness, goodness, and responsibility; furthermore, the decision apparently cannot produce satisfactory outcomes for each value.

In case 1.1, the conflict is between Mr. Slawinski's (and the therapist's) desire to continue his rehabilitation to normal life and the need to protect society and Mr. Slawinski himself against the risks of premature discharge. If you find yourself leaning toward the importance of safeguarding society and Mr. Slawinski himself because of the serious consequences of guessing wrong about his competence, you are probably using a common approach to ethical decision making called "consequentialism." If you find yourself thinking of ways to compromise between what Mr. Slawinski is asking for and the need to protect him and society against premature certification, this, too, is probably a consequentialist approach: you are trying to maximize good consequences and minimize bad ones.

In case 1.2, the main conflict is the need to respect the authority of patients and families to determine how they will be treated versus the need to treat potential transplant recipients fairly. If you find yourself feeling that there is something unfair about promoting the rock star to the head of the transplant list, you are probably reasoning according to principles, in this case the principle of fairness, the concept that similar cases ought to be treated similarly. If, however, you find yourself uncomfortable about withholding important information from responsible decision makers, you may be reasoning from the professional responsibility to promote patient and family autonomy. Most likely you feel some concern about both fairness and withholding relevant information, and therefore you may be unsure what would be professionally responsible in a case like this.

In case 1.3, the conflict involves the principle of nonabandonment and questions about disconnecting patients from life support versus considerations of social and monetary costs. Here all three perspectives come into play: reasoning from principles, consequences, and professional character (or virtue) pull thoughtful people in differing directions. While these ethical decision-making perspectives may not always come together easily, we will come to see that, in general, they can provide the most professionally responsible ways to make and explain the basis for ethical decisions.

Here are three more key ideas. Reasoning from principles *is ethical decision making guided by basic values (such as fairness), or professional values (such as not abandoning patients).* Consequentialism *is ethical decision making guided by the goal of achieving the best balance of good outcomes with the least sacrifice of important values.* Professional character, *or* virtue ethics, *is ethical decision making guided by such personal traits as loyalty, kindness, or integrity.*

The apparent conflicts in these cases are characteristic of ethical dilemmas, or problems. Dilemmas arise when competing values cannot all be satisfied. What makes these conflicts *ethical* dilemmas is that unless decisions about how to resolve these situations are perceived as fair, just, right or good, and responsible—that is "ethical"—by all the affected parties (including society as a whole), the result is likely to be perceived as ethically irresponsible or, more simply, "wrong" or "unethical." Note that not all the values at stake in an ethical dilemma have to be ethical ones to create an ethical problem. Financial values, religious values, legal values, political values, professional values, and institutional values—literally all kinds of values—can contribute to an ethical dilemma. What makes a dilemma an ethical one is not what kind of values are involved in the conflict, but whether the decision about how to resolve the problem will be held to standards of fairness, justice, rightness or goodness, and responsibility—that is, to ethical standards.[1]

Very roughly, *fairness* and *justice* are especially good examples of widely held ethical principles and correspond to what is often called deontological ethics, or reasoning from principles. *Rightness* or *goodness* are highly ambiguous terms: they are used in a host of ways. Here, they roughly correspond to judgments that a decision promotes a desirable or beneficial state of affairs. Such judgments are characteristic of teleological or consequentialist forms of ethical reasoning. The terms *responsible* or *professional* suggest that a decision lives up to values or traits of character that make up a model or ideal health care practitioner and are characteristic of virtue ethics. Each of these approaches to ethical decision making will be explored much more fully in later sections of this book.

This point—that ethics is not some limited or special collection of values or issues, but rather concerns the broadest spectrum of human decision making—is critically important.

> It is at the very heart of being human to recognize the importance of ethical ideas. These are the ideas we have about how relations between people can be, might be, ought to be. They are beliefs about how life ought to be lived; they are the interests and ideals that help us in shaping purposes of life that give meaning to the variety of ways human beings can interact with each other, with other species, and with the environment. Ethical thought consists in the orderly examination of these ideas, beliefs, interests, and ideals, as well as in raising new questions about them in the context of our own present circumstances. (Nyberg, 1993, p. 195)

From this perspective, it is clear that ethical issues in health care are not limited to the kinds of high-profile problems that attract public and media attention. Although most people probably think of abortion, euthanasia, assisted suicide, and the like as the ethical issues most central to health care, in fact issues of informed consent, whistle blowing, conflicting priorities, personal responsibility and integrity, health care access and cost, end-of-life decisions, and business practices are far more likely to occupy health care providers' time and concern.

---

[1] Each of these terms is likely to be understood in differing ways by different readers at this stage. In fact, defining them precisely is an issue philosophers debate seriously. For the moment, we can rely on an intuitive understanding that can be refined as we go along.

So, for the time being, let us adopt a rough-and-ready definition to be expanded later: ethics is the study and practice of responsibly resolving situations in which values or interests appear to conflict. Ethical theory, also called moral philosophy, is the effort to explain ethical reasoning in a comprehensive way. Ethical practice, as related to ethical theory, involves trying to resolve ethical conflicts and confusions by reference to interpersonally valid standards of reasoning and value. Whether there are such standards, whether all reasonable people at some level do accept similar standards of rationality and deep values (or would accept similar standards if they thought about it carefully), is an issue over which there is disagreement, and we examine it later.

For the moment, however, note that most ethical problems arising in health care involve more than one person and therefore require solutions that will be acceptable to more than one person. Moreover, as health care moves steadily in the direction of interdisciplinary, comprehensive case management, differing interests and priorities between departments will need to be addressed in ways that can be seen as fair, right, and responsible by all parties. Thus, languages and procedures for achieving the resolution of value or interest conflicts must go beyond personal or disciplinary lines. Philosophers strongly urge that such resolutions ought to be as mutually respectful as possible and note that when intimidation, political authority, or coercion is substituted for reasoning, respect for people and their interests is lost. In such circumstances, the results will typically appear unethical, especially to those whose interests are sacrificed.

Thus, the goal of ethical decision making is to attain mutually respected solutions to everyday conflicts between competing human values. Such decision making cannot prosper in an environment of disrespect for people, personal and professional intolerance, or closed-mindedness. It flourishes where genuine participatory decision making and mutual trust is widely practiced. Helping to create environments supportive of ethical decision making is itself an important ethical issue.

WHAT TO EXPECT FROM STUDYING ETHICS

Some people expect too much from studying ethics. Some expect too little. Studying ethics will not solve all the problems of health care, let alone all the important personal and social issues involving values. At the same time, studying ethics is not an abstract exercise far removed from important problems. If studying ethics were a matter of merely looking over some quaint historical ideas about values or merely wringing our hands and venting about how troubling some current events and practices are, then studying ethics would not be worth our time.

The study of ethics, or moral philosophy, has four goals. These are to develop sensitivity to issues involving conflicts among values, to develop fluent moral reasoning, to develop the ability to resolve value conflicts in ways that stand up to interpersonal scrutiny, and to encourage practices, policies, and institutions that reflect responsible ethical decision making. However ambitious these goals are, and they are very ambitious, some people are disappointed by them because they expect studying ethics to accomplish other purposes—such as making sure all health care professionals always demonstrate exemplary moral conduct in their personal as well as their professional lives, or providing a kind of encyclopedia of the right answers to ethical problems in health care. For better or worse, we cannot promise any such things.

Ethics is not the same as moral reform. Studying ethics should enable people to think more clearly and honestly about ethical matters, but putting their considered moral judgments into practice remains as difficult as always. Leading an ethical life requires the development of character, a project which, as many moral philosophers from many cultures have observed, is not only hard work, but also takes a whole lifetime of steady commitment. Additionally, ethics is not surrogate moral decision making. Studying ethics will not and should not provide anyone with a list of moral actions and decisions that will relieve them of the right and responsibility to make moral decisions, nor will it provide anyone with an ethical encyclopedia in which to look up the answers to moral dilemmas. Such an encyclopedia could never be complete enough to provide answers to all the questions people will encounter over their careers, nor is there any reason to suppose its answers would necessarily be valid or justified. (Some people may think that one of the functions of religion is to provide just this kind of guidance. But there are problems with this view, especially in the pluralistic world of contemporary health care, where many colleagues and clients will not share the same religious views. We will discuss this issue more fully in Chapter 2.)

Somewhat more controversially, our approach to ethics does not involve moral indoctrination. That is, as we approach it, studying and practicing ethics requires that all values and particular outcomes initially be treated with the same evenhanded critical examination. None is to be considered privileged from the start. So, for example, we do not start from the position that abortion is always morally wrong or that choice is always morally right and then reason in such a way as to prove our position. In this we differ from some approaches to ethics that start with certain positions on issues and make it the point of studying ethics to assure that others accept the "party line." We believe that if an approach or position really is authoritative, its authority will emerge from a fair and evenhanded evaluation of the alternatives. Moreover, we believe that students will be far better equipped to believe in and convince others of the positions they accept if they have arrived at them by a problem-solving process that includes fair consideration of the alternatives.

Finally, although our position is somewhat controversial, we do not sharply distinguish professional ethics from private morality. One reason is that we do not believe people's personal and professional lives can be tightly compartmentalized. Another is that we think there are professional ethical issues that overlap both public and private moral life. Further, we think a true professional is a morally sensitive and decent human being, not merely a shrewd calculator of consequences or a rigid follower of codes of professional ethics or other rules of conduct. Professional ethics is an inextricable part of a complete life. So, even if people could compartmentalize life into separate professional and private areas, the virtues of each one belong in the other as well: fairness, justice, mercy, and concern about good outcomes are equally important whether one is on the job or not.

We recognize that people may not agree about these questions. We think one reason to study ethics is to develop your own thoughtful positions on controversial issues.

QUESTIONS FOR DISCUSSION

1. Identify an ethical issue or problem you have had to face. What values or interests appeared to be in conflict? How did you resolve the problem? Did your solution work well? Why or why not?

2. We have suggested that there are probably some ethical values that are universally accepted (or would be if people thought about them carefully). What would be some examples? Or does the fact that some people disagree about some values show that there are no universally accepted values? Discuss.

3. Do you agree that a person's professional ethics also extend into a person's private life? Or do you think professional ethics are one thing, and a person's private life is something else entirely? Should people "practice what they preach" wherever they find themselves? Or is there an area of privacy in nonprofessional life where it's nobody's business what people do? Explain, using specific examples.

WHY ETHICS? AND WHY NOW?

The study of ethics by health care professionals is not a new phenomenon. In fact, throughout history, from Hippocrates, to the great tradition of health care in religious orders, to the work of Florence Nightingale, training in the practice of health care has been linked to moral and ethical considerations in an indissoluble bond. Yet emphasis on courses in health care ethics that take a philosophical approach, as well as the widespread establishment of institutional review boards (IRBs) or institutional ethics committees (IECs), is a fairly recent phenomenon, beginning in the 1970s.[2] There is little reason to think that health care practitioners suddenly became less ethical in the late twentieth century than they were when ethical attitudes and practices were studied along with other professional knowledge. So why the emphasis on ethics now?

Several issues have been especially influential in propelling the interest in ethics and IECs. One is a series of highly publicized court decisions concerning the end of life. Perhaps the most famous of these is the ruling of the New Jersey Supreme Court in 1976 that Karen Ann Quinlan's father could legally direct that her ventilator be turned off and other support be withdrawn and that legal immunity would be granted to physicians and the hospitals involved. The court also suggested but did not require that any further such cases could be resolved by hospital ethics committees. So, almost immediately, hospitals and long-term-care facilities had a strong reason to establish IECs: the possibility that they would have to deal with cases like Quinlan's. But, of course, the Quinlan case did not occur in an ethical vacuum. End-of-life cases stir profound ethical anxieties among health professionals. The problems become much more common and acute as technology, such as the ventilator and other forms of life support used by Quinlan's physicians, prolongs dying. So a combination of advancing technology and court decisions contributes to end-of-life ethical interests.

Perhaps it is unnecessary to do more than mention the parallel concerns at the beginning of life. As technology has made possible the survival of infants born with severe defects, serious questions arise about

---

[2] We prefer the term "institutional ethics committee," or IEC, to the term "institutional review board," or IRB, for several reasons. In our experience, the most effective institutional ethics committees are not confined to retrospective analysis of problem cases, or "review," but also anticipate problems and issues so they can advise on ways to avoid them. Moreover, IRBs are often associated with the specific task of evaluating research proposals and/or patient care issues, while IECs can address broader issues in which ethical elements appear. This is a model we advocate, and this broader role is reflected in cases we discuss, notably in Chapter 4.

whether all such lives should be saved at any cost. But if not, how does one draw an ethical line with any confidence?

The Human Genome Project, an international effort to map traits and disease "sites" in human DNA, is another example of technology propelling ethical concerns. While genetic research has disclosed many markers for disease conditions, little progress has been made in prevention or cure of those conditions. Do people who are genetically at risk for diseases have any obligation to verify their risks through testing? Do they have any obligation to inform others, such as their spouses or potential spouses? Do they have any obligation at least to consider their potential for passing on "defective" genes to offspring before they have children? Are there any disease conditions so bad that it would be wrong to conceive or to bear children who have the genetic preconditions for those diseases? These are just a few of the issues created by genetic technology.

Another ethical influence of a more pervasive kind is a series of problems concerning allocation of resources. When kidney dialysis machines first became available in the 1960s and early 1970s, they were scarce and expensive, and opportunities for their use had to be rationed among competing applicants. Selection committees, composed of doctors and community leaders, set up their own (sometimes widely differing) criteria for choice; these committees, in turn, provoked spirited ethical debate and metamorphosed into IECs. In 1972, Congress alleviated the problem by funding dialysis for virtually everyone who needs it. But, in this era of tighter and tighter health care funding, allocation problems continue, not only in areas of exotic therapies, such as organ transplants, but even—and increasingly—in the area of day-to-day priority decisions. Thus the combination of increasingly complex and costly care and limitations on both financial and other resources (such as the absolute scarcity of organs for transplantation) creates additional ethical pressures.

Other kinds of resource allocation problems exist—for example, in research and development. New drugs must be tested for effectiveness and safety. But those tests will normally involve subjecting some people (or animals) to significant risks, while depriving others (the "control group") of what may be their only hope, an experimental breakthrough. And, given that so many health care needs are still unmet, how much of the finite health care budget should be put into research? Should politics steer research in desired directions? Or should market forces be allowed to direct attention to projects that promise rapid payoffs?

In sum, two aspects of modern life that give rise to ethical concerns are rapid changes in technology and problems of resource allocation, especially when combined with various forms of social concern (such as cost containment, access, and social justice issues) and professional oversight. New technologies create allocation problems because they are often in limited supply and expensive. But they also raise questions about how or whether to use the new technology and how to steer it in responsible directions.

In addition to these technological and resource allocation issues, today there are also considerations internal to the professional practices of health care providers. Regardless of specialty, health care professionals are experiencing increasing responsibility and accountability to peers, the public, internal review agencies, government agencies, and so forth. It is not an exaggeration to say that virtually nothing done by any health care professional goes unreviewed by someone. Accordingly, there is a growing need for a sense of what the ethical parameters of decisions are, so that they will survive external review.

> The Joint Commission on Accreditation of Health Care Organizations (JCAHO) specifies the standards health care institutions must meet to be eligible to serve the public. The JCAHO requires that ethics committees or people in a similar role be available to help resolve and review ethical dilemmas. The JCAHO standards also address patient rights and organizational responsibilities and require that hospitals and other institutions make provisions to cover issues such as patient preferences in care, informed consent, and family participation in care decisions as well as ensure that business is conducted according to a responsible code of ethical behavior (Joint Commission, 1998).

Another kind of professional concern arises when there are conflicts between personal, professional, and societal values and expectations. Among these are situations in which low staffing, sicker patients, and stress conflict with people's need to maintain a perspective and balance between their personal and professional lives. Many health professionals become uncomfortable with all the ways in which contemporary practice seems to let patients "slip through the the cracks" or otherwise disregards patients' priorities; an example is the routine violation of confidentiality and privacy that occurs in hospitals.

> Historically, health care ethics has emphasized the two values of confidentiality and privacy. Florence Nightingale (1859) said of confidentiality, "And remember every nurse should be one who is depended upon, in other words, capable of being a 'confidential' nurse. She must be no gossip, no vain talker; she should never answer questions about her sick except to those who have a right to ask them" (p. 70). Consider, however, how many people, from patient admission through discharge and reimbursement from the third-party payer, not to mention the family of the person in the next bed, have access to the details of a patient's situation, yet have no real need for that information.

Society creates other pressures. Widely publicized instances of corporate, individual, and professional irresponsibility foster an intense public sense of outrage, with a corresponding demand that new emphasis be placed on ethics. Meanwhile, however, there is also a widespread loss of confidence in professional institutions, such as hospitals, which once enjoyed an almost complete public trust. (Just why such institutions as hospitals have lost public trust is a complicated question in which unreasonable public expectations, high costs, management according to business rather than public service models, personnel problems, and other factors all play a part.) It is also true that, as health care institutions become more bureaucratic, the public feels an increasing sense of powerlessness due to the complexity, impersonality, and sometimes inhumane quality of institutions, as well as the increasing specialization of service providers. The lack of information provided to patients, combined with the amazingly intrusive invasions of privacy that are preconditions for receipt of services, is also very troubling.

As already mentioned, another important societal concern is cost. With health care consuming 14 percent of the American gross domestic product (GDP), with ever-increasing co-pays, fewer jobs that include comprehensive benefits, unaffordable private health insurance, and higher taxes and cost-shifting for those unable to pay, many people in American society feel more and more certain that there is something profoundly unjust about American health care; and people are more and more bitterly resentful of the frustrations involved in dealing with health problems. Often that resentment is expressed by society's unwillingness to pay adequately for the care of those whom it sees as less valuable (for example, the elderly or those receiving public assistance) or those whom it sees as irresponsible.

And there are ethical pressures that develop over time in the hearts and minds of health care practitioners. These internal pressures include a growing sense of hopelessness and meaninglessness, a sense that, as professionals sometimes say, "We're only putting Band-Aids on the problems," which are, it seems, always getting worse. Like society as a whole, health professionals recognize the lack of moral consensus that surrounds us all and a sense that many traditional sources of moral guidance are ineffective or untrustworthy. Indeed, the impersonality and sterility of many events and activities in daily life create a sense that things are not as they should be, a sense that somehow morality and public community have been eroded in ways that leave us with less fulfilling and less humane lives.

Furthermore, health care providers and recipients are members of a pluralistic society. As our global community expands, it is not uncommon for providers and patients alike to be of differing ethnic, cultural, and social backgrounds. Living in a world of pluralistic values sometimes creates a sense of despair, a feeling that there is nothing left to hold on to. It can also create the fear that with so many differing values, consensus can never be achieved. In fact, however, resolving ethical dilemmas responsibly becomes even more critical because of diverse human values.

It is, of course, asking too much to expect that any study of ethics will meet all these demands or relieve all these pressures. Still, the need to address them does help explain why emphasis is now being placed on professional ethics in health care.

ETHICAL ISSUES: NORMATIVE AND MOTIVATIONAL

In spite of the many factors contributing to a heightened sense of the importance of ethical issues, ethical dilemmas ultimately resolve into only two fundamental types of questions: "What is the right thing to do?" and "Why do the right thing once I know what it is?" The first of these is called a "normative" ethical question, a question about how we know what would be ethically responsible or the right thing to do. The second of these is a "motivational" question because it concerns how to get someone to act ethically. That there are motivational questions draws attention to a fact noted earlier, that studying ethics, or even taking a thoughtful position on an issue, is not the same thing as acting ethically, nor is it any sort of guarantee. To understand the difference more clearly, consider the examples that follow.

Case 1.4: Severe Birth Defects Versus Aggressive Care

Baby H is born with physical and cosmetic abnormalities so profound as to leave very little (but not zero) probability that he can live longer than a few weeks, even with extensive (and expensive) life support and surgical intervention. His mother seems not to understand the situation; no other family is available; and it appears highly unlikely the hospital can recoup more than 40 percent of its costs. Should Baby H be treated aggressively?

Case 1.5: Professional Responsibility Versus Family Obligation

Alice P. is an oncology nurse on an understaffed unit. She is also a supportive mom and a big fan of her daughter Jenny's ballet performances. Alice has used up all her personal leave time escorting Jenny to performances and competitions; and, in fact, she has called in ill in order to help Jenny's career when Alice's supervisor has been unable to grant additional leave. Jenny has been very successful; she's auditioning next week for the role of Clara in *The Nutcracker*. Unable to find anyone to cover for her, and unable to take any more leave time, Alice realizes that she can probably get away with calling in ill a few more times before serious disciplinary measures come into play. Should she call in ill?

Morally sensitive, conscientious people are likely to differ over how to treat Baby H. But there is no serious difficulty in knowing what the ethically responsible thing for Alice to do is. Calling in ill is straightforwardly dishonest, as well as unfair to her employer, her coworkers, and her patients; therefore, she shouldn't call in. Nevertheless, the temptation for Alice to behave unethically in this situation may be strong indeed. And, as anyone who has worked in health care knows, it happens all the time.

In part because her obligation is so clear and the temptation is so strong, Alice may feel she ought to avoid the shame or guilt of behaving unethically by trying to redescribe the situation in a way that is more favorable to her and also excuses her unethical behavior. For example, she may feel that the ungenerous personnel policies of her employer put otherwise conscientious people like her in a position where they have to lie. Another common, but equally dishonest, strategy is to camouflage her motivational problem as a normative conflict between principles. For example, instead of confronting her temptation to call in even though she has no ethical basis for doing so, she might try to justify her actions on the grounds that "My obligations as a parent come before my obligations to my job," which is a judgment many people might agree with. And Alice might really believe this too. But in this instance, given the way her reasoning is described in case 1.5, she would be rationalizing her decision after the fact. To see how self-deceptive this is, we only need to note all the other ways she could fulfill her obligations as a parent and as an employee that do not involve lying to her employer.

> *What do you think about how Baby H ought to be treated? What are your reasons for thinking this? What about Alice? What are some other ways she could fulfill her responsibilities both as a supportive parent and as a conscientious employee?*

Studying ethics normally emphasizes normative problems and how to resolve them responsibly. This is because motivational problems—getting people to do the right thing when they don't want to—are not usually a matter of figuring out how best to resolve a conflict among interests and values; motivational problems are mostly a matter of getting people to set their interests aside when other interests clearly have a higher importance. Our own interests are powerful incentives: we frequently act so as to further our own wants, desires, and needs.

And yet there are circumstances in which doing the ethically responsible thing involves no benefit to ourselves or, even worse, involves compromising our own interests (or at least some of them). Consider the next case.

Case 1.6: Incompetence of a Colleague

Janice Newcombe, D.D.S., is a specialist in dental surgery and reconstructive dentistry, and she has gradually built up a strong reputation as the referral dentist of choice in her part of the state. Over the last several years, she has had a number of cases from Dr. Ben Alta, the only primary dentist in a small, rural town, who is nearing retirement. Many of the cases Dr. Alta has referred to Dr. Newcombe have involved what she considers sloppy work—inadequate cleaning and preparation for fillings, for example, which were also poorly installed and sealed and which therefore became problems again. But the cases Newcombe gets from Alta are also invariably interesting, complicated, and well reimbursed, especially in comparison to the rest of her client load. Does she have any ethical obligation to report Alta to the Board for disciplinary action?

The problem Dr. Newcombe faces is complicated by the fact that it is in her self-interest not to have Alta disciplined. If she were to initiate action against Alta, he would probably stop referring cases to her; and, if he were prevented from practicing (though this is not likely), residents of the small town he serves would have no care available to them locally. Moreover, Alta does send on those patients he becomes concerned about, and Newcombe is able to repair the damage, normally without arousing any suspicion in the patients that anyone has been incompetent or negligent. Dr. Newcombe likes these cases because they challenge her talents and skills, but also because they pay well. Yet, obviously, the patients are harmed, and so are those—patients or third-party payers—who have to pay for the "clean up" of Alta's poor practice. So, regardless of any benefits to her, it seems clear that Newcombe's professional ethical obligation is to act to stop Alta from practicing beyond his abilities. Even so, it should come as no surprise that Newcombe might try to address the issue in such a manner that her relationship with Dr. Alta is not upset.

> *Many seemingly normative ethical issues turn out to be motivational— situations where it's clear what the right thing to do is, but that right thing is something people don't want to do. Can you think of situations in your own experience where you knew what you ought to have done but didn't or wouldn't do it?*

SUMMING UP: WHAT WE KNOW
ABOUT ETHICS SO FAR

As people experience them, ethical issues typically involve apparent conflict among values or interests, not all of which are necessarily ethical values. Much ethical conflict pits moral values against legal, religious, institutional, or financial values. Any issue about which questions of fairness, justice, rightness or goodness, or professional responsibility can be raised is an ethical issue. And this means that virtually any decision or action that affects someone else, and many that affect only oneself, will have ethical dimensions.

Ethical issues always involve the need to choose responsibly, not on the basis of arbitrary or individual feelings without regard for others' interests. Such responsibility is often stressful, especially when decision makers lack some relevant information (which is most of the time), or when they have some personal or professional relationship with those whose interests or values conflict, or when the issue can have far-reaching consequences. When, in addition to trying to resolve the question "What is the right thing to do?" (normative), one also has to ask "How does one get people to do the right thing?" (motivational), it is easy to understand why many people find ethical issues uncomfortable.

So, the most common initial response to ethical problems is probably stress. People often deal with this stress by denial—either by not recognizing the problem as a problem or by trying to move the problem elsewhere, so it is not their problem, but someone else's. Sometimes, too, this evasion of responsibility takes the form of an effort to turn ethical issues into something that may appear easier to handle: practice problems, questions that can be resolved by factual research, legal problems, labor-management relations issues, and the like. For this reason, as well as to "map" the idea of ethics more clearly, we can refine our sense of what morality is and how it is often evaded by contrasting morality with other institutions. The most important of these are discussed in Chapter 2. Meanwhile, it's important to remember what studying ethics can and cannot do. It can guide responsible decision making. But it can't provide all the answers, it can't substitute for the moral courage it takes to act responsibly, it can't relieve people of their ethical responsibilities, or insulate people's lives from professional and personal accountability.

WHY MULTIDISCIPLINARY ETHICS?

All this discussion goes some way toward explaining why pressure for greater study and practice of professional ethics cannot be met by simply intensifying the study of professional values—unless a truly interdisciplinary perspective is taken. In the current environment of public concern and multidisciplinary—team-based—practice, professional ethics cannot simply be reduced to separate disciplines trying to impose their values on their members and on each other. They, and we, must learn to resolve problems together. Focusing too much on values and priorities internal to a discipline, values that may not be shared by members of other disciplines, can be part of the problem rather than part of the solution. The values of finance may not be the values of nursing, the values of hospice/home care may not be the values of the oncology department, the values of hospital legal counsel may not be the values of the public health department, and so it goes. Some standpoint independent of any particular health care discipline but common to all of them seems therefore to be the best hope for multidisciplinary professional ethics.

> Health care organizations have traditionally divided care by specialty. Unfortunately, when providers do not see beyond their departments, specialties, and disciplines, patients tend to "fall through the cracks." Effective continuity of care requires that health care providers join together as teammates to provide holistic patient services. This team approach is encouraged by credentialing agencies, who facilitate the team approach through an integration of disciplines in the standards of organizational performance. A parallel problem arises when ethical issues are segregated by departments, specialties, and disciplines. That is, important values tend to "fall through the cracks." Accordingly, conscientious health care agencies and credentialing organizations encourage a multidisciplinary, integrated approach to ethical problem solving.

A philosophical approach to ethics offers the recognition that most significant ethical problems are social, so that personal, individual solutions without reference to the interests and views of others are inadequate. Philosophy is unique in not assuming a privileged moral theory; it subjects all views to analysis by means of interpersonally valid criteria of rationality. Philosophy is not coercive, allowing individual response within a framework of rational consensus building. Philosophers emphasize that many difficult ethical problems have their roots in conceptual confusions and inaccuracies or problems in reasoning, and philosophy offers techniques to resolve such problems. Finally, the goal of philosophical professional ethics is to develop a process and acquire the skills necessary to resolve moral problems in ways that are as satisfactory as possible to all concerned, rather than to impose some arbitrary external judgment on beleaguered health professionals.

But a note of caution is in order here. Philosophy is not without significant drawbacks as a guide for professional ethical study of issues in health care. Philosophers must be careful not to become judges, looking down on those whose professional decisions do not meet philosophical standards of rigorous justification. Philosophers generally lack the clinical expertise of health professionals, as well as direct experience. So philosophers must resist the temptation to misconstrue their logical and theoretical sophistication as licenses to practice health care. What is needed here, as in so many other areas of life, is respectful collaboration.

QUESTIONS FOR DISCUSSION

1. What are some examples of new technologies that create ethical dilemmas? What, exactly, are the ethical problems they create?

2. How do you think that Dr. Newcombe should deal with the problem presented by Dr. Alta's patients? What values are coming into conflict here? What are three or four alternatives she should consider? Which is the best choice? Why?

3. Have you had troubling experiences with any aspect of the American health care system? What were they? What made them an ethical problem? What could or should have been done about them?

4. *Case 1.7: Uncomfortable Working Relationship*—Carolyn, a nurse with two years of experience on her unit, observes a conversation between Martha, the most senior nurse on the unit, and Ginger, a nurse who has recently completed orientation, but who has little experience. Ginger has asked Martha for some guidance in handling a clinical situation she has not seen before, and Martha tells her what to do—but her information is wrong. Not wanting to embarrass Martha or become the target of Martha's famous temper, Carolyn resolves to straighten things out with Ginger later on. Are there any ethical issues involved in this situation? Are there normative ones? Motivational ones? How should situations like this be handled?

CHAPTER TWO

Comparisons and Contrasts: Ethics and Other Matters

HOW DO WE KNOW WHAT IS THE RIGHT THING TO DO?

In this chapter, we explore relations between ethical decision making and a number of substitutes people sometimes use to avoid the difficulties of genuine moral reasoning. These substitutes include role fulfillment, feelings, law, religion, human rights, professional codes and oaths, and current standards of practice. While these substitutes are valid concepts in and of themselves, they are not necessarily based on responsible ethical principles. People use them as substitutes because these concepts do shape our thinking and contribute to our decision making on other grounds. But personal validity is different from ethical responsibility.

FULFILL YOUR ROLE

One common approach to "ethical" decision making that, as we will see, is ultimately unsatisfactory is to fulfill one's job description, or role, and nothing more. While assuming a professional role is one way for the novice practitioner to become acculturated into a profession, role fulfillment is not intended to be the sole means by which decisions are made, especially for the experienced professional. However, this approach is consistent with the tradition mentioned earlier, that one absorbs the ethics of one's profession by practicing it. Consider, however, the following case.

Case 2.1: Rigid Definition of Role

Katherine M., R.N., B.S.N., works the 11:00 P.M. to 7:00 A.M. shift on a medical surgical unit, along with two nursing assistants and an L.P.N. Although all of them are seldom busy at once, Katherine is

21

very selective about what she takes on and is sometimes simply unwilling to help the others with what she considers mundane or routine activities. Tonight, when Katherine and one of the nursing assistants, Lucinda, were behind the desk, two call lights went off at once. Heading toward one room, Lucinda asked, "You want to get room 14?" Katherine replied, "Nah. That's just a potty run. I didn't go to college just to help people to the john." Is Katherine's behavior unethical (professionally irresponsible)?

Each person plays many roles; examples include spouse, parent, employee, driver, and student. The list can be long and each role imposes certain responsibilities typical of specific relationships: fidelity, care of one's children, fulfilling work expectations, observing traffic laws, doing homework, and so on. Some writers have suggested that ethics, especially professional ethics, may just be the sum of one's obligations as a professional. (They sometimes distinguish between these ethical obligations and personal morality.) A special case of this approach is the emphasis placed in health care education on defining the various roles of members of the health care team. Defining roles is important in delineating responsibility for specific interventions and clarifying these responsibilities between health care team members. One must not become locked strictly into position descriptions, performance expectations, and definitions of scope of practice. Instead, the idea is to internalize the intent of the professional role.

Role confusion is common in health care. Defining roles is important because it identifies who is really responsible for a specific task or activity. But, because responsibilities overlap, some responsibilities may be neglected because one provider believes that another provider is following through.

Problems also arise when one's professional role is defined too narrowly—perhaps to avoid unwanted tasks. Other problems arise because the criteria for what counts as a role, or what obligations go with what roles, may have no direct relationship with conscientiousness, competence, or skills. For example, one may have completed a B.S.N. degree, yet be lazy, unable to get along with people, or even clinically incompetent. The same dilemma can occur because subordinates may be more professional in important respects than their supervisors. It is likely that these sorts of tensions underlie the problems in case 2.1.

Further problems arise because role definition and expectations are not generally negotiated with other affected parties, nor are they often understood by those other affected parties. Coworkers tend to form expectations based on their experiences, not on a discipline's role definitions; patients generally have no understanding of the differences in roles between various health care providers and find the whole matter a frustrating evasion. (Whose responsibility is it to discuss medications with patients? The physician's? The nurse's? The pharmacist's? The discharge planner's? But if none of these people see it as their role, who suffers?)

In any event, disciplinary outsiders—patients and colleagues from other departments and health care fields, for example—may tend to develop role expectations different from those of insiders. Many patients find the differing roles and responsibilities of health care providers unintelligible, assuming instead that anyone in a white coat has the expertise to address any and all issues of concern to them. Directing issues to others is often seen as evasiveness, lack of cooperation, laziness, or lack of concern about patients' well-being.

Role responsibilities are separate from attitudes, skills, and actions associated with a role. Role responsibilities are not usually negotiated with other affected parties nor articulated effectively to those same parties. Thus, members of a professional group may or may not have a common understanding of what they should reasonably expect from their membership. And, because intraprofessional confusion occurs, interprofessional confusion should be expected. When ethics is reduced to roles alone, the result will inevitably produce tensions.

Of course, it cannot be professionally responsible to take on activities outside one's area of competence. Nevertheless, the biggest problem about role-based ethics is that defining one's role narrowly can be a way to evade legitimate responsibilities. "It's not in my job description" can serve as an excuse to avoid confronting difficult or unwanted issues. Now, having said this, it is important to recognize that roles and role-based responsibilities are an indispensable tool in health care. Teams are not constructed of people who all have the same responsibilities; instead, the fulfillment of various role-based responsibilities makes for the kind of smooth and effective teamwork that is essential in health care. The point is only that not all of one's ethical decisions can be dictated by adhering to one's role as a health care professional. The requirements of one's role should be considered a minimum standard of practice at best, and certainly not all that one needs to do or be to be professionally responsible.

And, finally, look back at cases 1.1 through 1.7. Would role-based ethics help resolve them? On the contrary, some of the cases we have considered become ethically problematic because aspects and values inherent in one's role are in conflict with each other.

FOLLOW YOUR FEELINGS

Another common, but deeply flawed, approach to "ethical" decision making is to consult one's own feelings. According to this approach, the right thing to do would be whatever one felt was right. This course of behavior has much intuitive appeal. But consider this case.

Case 2.2: Feelings Leading to Unprofessional Practice

Rosa M., L.P.N., is a profoundly conservative, religious person who strongly feels that homosexuality is a voluntary perversion forbidden by God. Her feelings on this issue are so strong, in fact, that she feels an almost physical aversion to those whom she suspects of being homosexual. While she recognizes (intellectually) that observance of universal precautions will reduce her risk of HIV infection to near zero, she advocates required disclosure of HIV status for patients who might be homosexual. She also feels staff should have a right of conscientious refusal where HIV patients are concerned. Is she ethically justified in these claims?

Some writers have emphasized the role of feelings, conscience, or intuition in ethical decision making. And, most likely, basing one's ideas on feelings is common not only in health care, but also in our culture generally. However, feelings by themselves are often unhelpful and even counterproductive to the resolution of moral problems. First, one needs to remember that ethical dilemmas are essentially conflicts in values. Often conflict among feelings is exactly the moral dilemma one has to face. Since one's feelings conflict, it is not very useful to try to use one's feelings to determine what is morally the best answer. Essentially, this would involve using conflicting feelings to mediate between conflicting values. In addition, feelings can be counterproductive because people's feelings can be unduly influenced by highly personal, perhaps inappropriate, factors (such as racism, sexism, homophobia); certainly most people would consider a racist's judgments to be unethical no matter how deeply the racist feels his hatred of others.

What are feelings? Feelings are emotions and attitudes people experience based on their perceptions of reality. In American culture, feelings are considered important as a basis for actions. In terms of ethics, feelings may guide actions, but they are not always wise guides. Further, while feelings may contribute to human values, feelings are not values. Rather, what we value influences our feelings. For example, if we value honesty, we will feel outrage when someone deliberately deceives us. So feelings are connected to values and to ethics, but they are not the same.

While feeling "comfortable" with the outcome is one desirable goal of moral decision making, not feeling comfortable does not by itself invalidate a decision. In some respects, comfort has little to do with an ethical decision because the very act of reaching a resolution between conflicts in values propels us into uncharted territory where much is new rather than comfortably familiar. Indeed, we are apt to find ourselves in situations where there are only better or worse—but not unambiguously good—choices; in those situations, when some important values have to be sacrificed, there may be no way to feel comfortable with the outcome. Besides, if, like Rosa, your feelings are not obviously ethical, the decision that "feels right" will actually be ethically questionable. Additionally, note that others—for example, the AIDS patients Rosa is so uncomfortable with—are unlikely to see Rosa's feelings as providing a persuasive justification for discriminating against them. This point applies generally. Quite simply, others normally do not accept "I felt like it" as a good reason to treat them in ethically questionable ways.

Finally, again, look back on the cases we have discussed so far. Would consulting one's feelings help solve any of them? In fact, it is precisely our conflicting feelings in most of these cases that contributes to the awkwardness and discomfort they provoke in most of us.

Again, this discussion is not intended to suggest that feelings are unimportant or that there is no appropriate role for feelings in ethics. We have already emphasized that increasing sensitivity to ethical issues is important. And, in fact, people who are unable to feel outrage at gross injustice or sympathy at suffering are, at the least, insensitive and perhaps even morally undeveloped. Feelings are ethically important because they goad us into action. And feelings (of shame, for example) are also important in helping us accept responsibility for our own actions. The point is that feelings by themselves are not very good guides to ethically responsible decision making.

OBEY THE LAW

Among the most frequently mentioned concerns health care professionals voice is their fear of malpractice suits. In this lawsuit-crazy society, it has become normal practice to ask legal counsel to review policies and procedures, press releases, labor negotiations, and management decisions precisely to avoid liability. Further, it has become very common to have counsel review and, in some cases, overrule institutional ethics committees, again to avoid any risk of increased liability. So common are practices like these that consulting the law increasingly substitutes for ethical decision making. But this approach, too, is not very satisfactory from the perspective of professional ethics.

Case 2.3: Patient Autonomy Versus Legal Limits

Consistent with state and federal funding legislation, staff at the St. Mary's Women's Health Clinic are not permitted to "counsel or suggest abortion" to any of their patients. Marianne B., however, believes that women have a moral right to explore all of their options; and, though she generally opposes abortion, she believes that, in some tragic cases, abortion may actually be the best (or least-bad) choice. She is currently counseling someone who may fit this description, a 14-year-old girl who is carrying a fetus with severe defects and whose own physical and mental health are very likely to be seriously compromised by continuing her pregnancy. Would Marianne be acting unethically by breaking the federal mandate (law) and discussing abortion with her client?

It is sometimes tempting to identify moral obligations with legal ones. However, these two concepts do not cover the same conduct. Laws are not always based on ethical considerations, so it is possible to violate a law without being immoral (some tax, zoning, and traffic laws may be like this), and it is also possible to behave unethically without violating a law (lying to customers, for example). At the same time, complying with some laws makes it difficult to behave ethically. For example, providing patients with adequate pain control could be considered to be at the borderline of illegality, since it is not legal to assist or appear to assist someone to commit suicide. At the same time, not providing adequate pain control to patients is unethical and unprofessional. Additionally, certain controlled substances have been found to be effective in managing pain and other symptoms, but it is illegal to possess or distribute them (marijuana, for example). Legal prohibitions are coercively sanctioned in ways that ethical norms are not; those who break a law are subject to arrest and punishment, but behaving unethically usually results in shame or guilt rather than fines and jail time. Accordingly, ethics is the broader concept, covering behavior considered right or wrong, good or bad, but not necessarily the kind of thing for which people will be punished.

Some people look hopefully to the law, the courts, to resolve difficult moral issues, often because they have no confidence in moral reasoning or public debate. Unfortunately, law often, even usually, follows consensus rather than creates it. So if there is no agreement on problematic issues, legislatures are often reluctant to act or courts to accept jurisdiction. When they do act or accept jurisdiction, however, legislatures and courts are as likely as anyone else to make morally obtuse or indefensible decisions. Furthermore, legal mechanisms are expensive, time-consuming, and frustrating. In addition, there are genuine questions about whether governments should be in the business of coercing some people to accept other people's ethical views. Many people like Marianne argue that some efforts to outlaw abortion reflect government (legal) intrusion into what is properly an individual moral decision.

The Michigan legislature's efforts to stop the activities of Dr. Jack Kevorkian while allowing compassionate end-of-life care nicely illustrate the points of our discussion. In 1994, the legislature set up a Commission on Death and Dying to recommend policy on assisted suicide. The commission deadlocked, splitting along the same lines as the general public. Meanwhile, Kevorkian assisted more than 100 suicides, often in gruesome, attention-grabbing ways. For four years, the legislature debated what to do; four efforts were made to prosecute Kevorkian, to no avail. In 1998, the legislature made assisting a suicide a felony, while at the same time a public referendum was being held to legalize a form of aid in dying. Even though a large majority of Michigan citizens favored aid in dying, they voted down the referendum. Meanwhile, after four efforts to prosecute Kevorkian had failed, he was finally convicted of second-degree murder (but not of assisting a suicide) in 1999.

In any event, under certain circumstances, people may be morally obligated to break laws. For example, it seems reasonable that those who broke laws to protect the lives of Jews during the Third Reich behaved morally in doing so. The same is true of many civil rights efforts during the 1950s and 1960s. And some people feel that assisting in active euthanasia may, in some situations, be another example. But as the assisted-suicide debate shows, there is no consensus on this issue.

Finally, once more, consider the cases we have discussed so far. Would consulting the law resolve any of them? It is not illegal for Katherine to avoid answering a call light nor is it illegal for Rosa to have her personal biases. It takes only a little thought to realize that the law is silent on all of the issues raised in the case studies. It is fair to say that the law is an important instrument for regulating social order and government policy. In fact, the law is "a system of principles and rules devised by organized society for the purpose of controlling human conduct" (Southwick, 1978). Its purpose is to provide a mechanism for dealing with conflicts between "individuals and government and those governed" (Southwick, 1979). But it is neither comprehensive enough, nor wise enough, to guide ethical decision making by itself. Moreover, there is an important role for pressures less coercive than legal sanctions—something moral judgments provide. Also, governments sometimes enact bad laws: laws that cannot be justified on moral grounds, such as those that enforced racism. In the cases of such laws, it might actually be morally wrong to obey the law. Of course, no conscientious, ethically sensitive person should recommend breaking a law without a very strong justification. Justifications for breaking laws ordinarily need to be unambiguous and powerful to be morally acceptable. But there can be ethical justifications for breaking unjust or unreasonably intrusive or restrictive laws. So, for all these reasons, legal considerations alone are not a substitute for ethical deliberation.

QUESTIONS FOR DISCUSSION

1. *Case 2.4: Role Conflicts Create Job Difficulties*—John C., R.N., B.S., nursing manager for the trauma center, is assisted by three coordinators. Of these, two are currently working on B.S.N. degrees part-time at a nearby college, while the third, Mary J., who already had completed a B.S.N. before moving to the area, has now finished her M.S.N. While her colleagues have extensive trauma care experience, Mary does not; her clinical background is primarily in well-baby care. Tensions arise between Mary and her colleagues when Mary neglects responsibilities she associates with subordinate roles in favor of activities that she associates with her master's-prepared role. (Her colleagues see her as condescending when she does this.) Mary also makes decisions for the department without consulting either her colleagues or her nursing manager.
    It has now come to John's attention that Mary has not yet begun a series of chart audits that John needs for a trauma department meeting the next day. When asked, Mary says she has spent the past two days drawing up extremely detailed orientation schedules for newly hired B.S.N. staff, emphasizing "transition to the trauma nurse role." Mary further points out that whereas her colleagues could do the chart audits (if they had time), only a master's-prepared nurse could provide orientation for the new staff. She feels offended that John is clearly unhappy with her performance. Is Mary behaving unethically? How should this problem be addressed?

2. Most students would probably agree that refusing to treat someone because of feelings of racism or sexism or homophobia is inconsistent with professionalism. How would your thinking about

the relevance of feelings to ethical decision making change (if at all) if Rosa refused to accept assignments to assist in abortion cases because of her strong anti-abortion feelings? If you see a difference between these cases, explain what it is. What about the potential for a "slippery slope" problem: that if we grant conscientious exemptions based on some feelings, we may have to grant exemptions based on other feelings, no matter what they are?

3. Operators of adult foster care facilities recently received a letter from the state's department of social services. The letter advised that, regardless of advance directives, participation in hospice, or standing no-code orders, staff must immediately call 911 in the event that a patient experienced any life-threatening episode or dangerous incident. In a discussion with the institutional ethics committee of the corporation that managed a number of such facilities, staff indicated they did not feel they could ethically comply with this law, because it went directly against their clients' stated wishes, as well as violating their own commitment to the values of hospice. One staff person said, "Well, if I do have to call, I'm not going to be in any rush to get to the telephone, that's for sure." But the corporate risk manager was livid. "If you break the law," she insisted, "you not only put yourself at risk, but you also violate your obligation to this corporation—you should be fired!" How does this case illustrate problems between ethical and legal values? Is there any way to reconcile the two? What do you think the staff ought to do when cases like this arise?

4. *Case 2.5: Prejudices Influence Facilities Scheduling*—Leah is the facilities manager for Campus Ridge Physician's Hospital, and she has been encouraged to try to market the group's meeting rooms, auditorium, and food services to outside organizations and agencies for meetings, seminars, and other events. Several business clubs are regular customers. But Leah has received a request from the Bay Area Gay and Lesbian Alliance to book the facilities. The dates the Alliance wants are open. But Leah is pretty sure that at least some of the business clubs would be uncomfortable enough about sharing facilities with the Alliance that they would choose another venue for their meetings. Leah is tempted to turn the Alliance down. Are any ethical issues involved in this situation? How should situations like this be handled? Would it make any difference if the group seeking to book the facilities were the Ku Klux Klan? Would it make any difference if the group were the regional smokers' rights organization?

FOLLOW YOUR RELIGIOUS BELIEF

One of the most common views of ethics holds that the only authoritative source for moral guidance is religious belief. "If God is dead, anything is permitted," said Dostoyevsky, and contemporary American political figures echo the idea by tracing the breakdown of public morality to the erosion of "traditional religious values." Is it, then, professionally responsible to locate ethics under the umbrella of religion?

Case 2.6: Religious Belief Versus Medical Care

David K. is a member of a fundamentalist Christian church that construes blood transfusions as violations of the biblical prohibitions against eating blood. His 12-year-old son Jonathan, who is unconscious as he arrives at the emergency room, will probably die if he is not transfused. Is it ethically (professionally) responsible to override David's religious morality and transfuse Jonathan?

In spite of the respect most people feel is due to serious religious convictions, virtually no health care providers would accept David's limitations on treating Jonathan. If safe and standard practice requires transfusion, and if there are no effective alternatives acceptable to David, they are likely to seek legal permission to appoint a temporary guardian for Jonathan who would authorize the transfusion. The ethical basis for this course of action is the idea that subjecting an incompetent minor to life-threatening risk because of convictions he may not share when he is fully able to think for himself does not constitute respecting the best interests of that minor. Perhaps, it is argued, only competent adults have the right kind of standing to make life-threatening choices, and then only for themselves or for other competent adults who have designated them as surrogates, whether or not their choice is guided by religious belief. What, then, is the best way to understand the relationship between religion and ethics in the context of health care?

Many people associate morality with religion. In fact, many people go so far as to say that unless morality is based on religion, morality has no validity or meaning. However, it seems possible to be a nonbeliever, yet lead a thoroughly moral life, at least by some widely accepted standards of morality. In addition, there are many different and conflicting religious traditions; and, although most insist that they alone have the authoritative understanding of God's will for humanity, it is not clear how to determine which religion (if any) is right about this or whether those who are not parties to a given tradition are or ought to be bound by its ideas. Any tradition is likely to seem obviously right to those who were brought up inside it, and other traditions may well seem just as obviously wrong. Since religious belief (often associated with ethnic biases) has been invoked to justify at least some behavior that is not morally defensible—genocide, for example, in Bosnia and Kosovo—it is not obvious that religious guidance should be taken uncritically.

In practice, it is also important to remember that "religious belief" includes a great deal more than mainstream Christianity and Judaism; the client population of even rural areas includes Muslims, Hindus, Amish, communal sectarians, Aryan supremacists, and others. So will the population of coworkers at virtually any health care institution. Since ethical practice decisions affect people on all sides of religious debates, it is important that the process by which they were arrived at be perceived as fair regardless of religious belief or lack of it. As a way of justifying ethical decisions, saying "I'm a Catholic, and we believe that abortion is always wrong, so it would be morally wrong for you to have an abortion" is unpersuasive to those who do not accept the authority of the Catholic Church, just as Islamic ideas are not persuasive to Jews or Hindus. Furthermore, not all of those who consider themselves to be Catholic do actually hold that abortion is always wrong, any more than all Muslims, Jews, or Hindus share the same moral views. So "according to my religion" offers no assurance that anyone else, even members of the same religious tradition, will necessarily accept the claims that follow.

However, according to many authorities within several otherwise divergent religious traditions, with enough careful thought and sympathetic understanding, the judgments of faith-based ethics and those of natural reason (or secular philosophy if it is properly conducted) will ultimately converge. That is, even if our own, personal ethical judgment was the result of inspiration through prayer, for example, there should be a rational justification independent of religious commitments that also can be articulated to justify our decisions to those who may not share a similar appreciation of religious inspiration.

In other words, religion supports ethical decision making, but cannot be the sole basis for ethical problem solving because not everyone shares identical religious beliefs. Ethical reasoning, however, levels the decision-making field because responsible ethical reasoning gives appropriate weight to people's religious values, while offering a respectful hearing for a diversity of other values. Often religious reasoning and ethical reasoning that is not specifically religious will converge on important issues.

Nonetheless, if our faith-based ethics conflict deeply with the best rational judgments we can make based on all the evidence and our best thinking, we may have an obligation to reconsider—or at least question—our religious convictions. After all, it might turn out that those religious convictions are being misunderstood or misinterpreted or even that the counsel they seem to suggest is really morally wrong. These are controversial claims explicitly opposed by some traditions. But if proper religious and secular moral reasoning do ultimately converge, this may constitute a kind of hope for resolving the apparently divisive moral differences among various religious traditions.

Once more, consider the cases we have explored so far. How many of them can be resolved in any straightforward way by consulting religious sources? Religious sources (as opposed to at least some of those who interpret them) seldom offer unambiguous guidance in the sorts of dilemmas that confront health care professionals. Perhaps it is not unfair to add that those who claim dogmatic certainty about what God's will is in every situation probably ought to inspire some caution among the rest of us. It is important to remember the distinction between religion and ethical decision making in health care where religious pluralism is represented across all health care disciplines.

None of this means religious belief need be irrelevant to people's moral lives. It remains true that religious belief is the source of many people's moral beliefs. And it is also true (and important) that religious belief can provide a powerful support for one's moral beliefs and efforts. Perhaps the expectation that religion will play an important role in health care ethics stems from the long and profoundly admirable tradition of religious orders in health care. However, it is important to remember the distinction between where someone's ethical judgments come from and what makes them acceptable in the context of health care practice—especially when religious pluralism is well represented across all health care disciplines. In terms of functioning ethically in a pluralistic, secular society, religious justifications for moral commitments often fail to provide a professionally defensible rationale for ethical judgments for two reasons. First, the religious commitments and assumptions on which they are based are not universally shared. Second, because they are not universally shared, ethical judgments influenced by religious beliefs require justifications that others will accept regardless of their religious commitments or lack of them. And these justifications usually will be most acceptable when they rely on secular patterns of reasoning and analysis.

RESPECT PEOPLE'S RIGHTS

One of the most common ways in which to describe ethical issues is in terms of the conflicting rights that may be involved. In fact, documents such as the "Patients' Bill of Rights" and codes of professional ethics are often framed in terms of rights. It is natural, then, for many people to think of ethical decision making primarily in terms of resolving priorities among rights. Consider the next case.

Case 2.7: Rights-Based Arguments and Abortion

Diane M. and Rachel F. disagree about the morality of abortion. Diane thinks the baby's right to life always overrides the mother's right to self-determination. Rachel denies that a fetus generally has rights as compelling as those of an adult woman, at least during the first two trimesters, and she thinks that under some unfortunate circumstances the rights of the mother have to override those of the fetus.

All parties to the abortion controversy will recognize arguments like this one: discussions are framed in terms of conflicts among rights. According to this approach, the morally appropriate course of action is the one that violates peoples' rights least or the one that preserves the highest-priority rights and sacrifices the lowest-priority rights. However, as this case shows, it is typically difficult to agree about which rights take priority over which, at least in many problematic cases. Here, for example, Diane and Rachel disagree about which right has the higher priority: self-determination or the baby's right to life. How does one "weigh" rights to decide which is more basic or fundamental or which ought to command the greatest respect? Effective ethical thinking should help decide this question, not deadlock over it.

It is also typically more difficult to decide who has what rights than it is to decide what is ethically responsible because the concept of rights is founded on the concept of what is morally right. Although philosophers disagree about exactly how to analyze the concept of rights, most would accept the idea that rights involve a "just claim." But the question of what constitutes a just claim or what justice requires is exactly a central question of what ethical responsibility requires. So, if we cannot tell who has what rights until we know whose claims are just, why not hold the discussion on the level of principles of justice rather than deciding what is just and then expressing the result in terms of rights?

What is a "just claim"? Justice is based on principles of equity, fairness, and integrity. Thus, someone with a just claim has an interest that must be recognized and accepted by others based on principles of equity, fairness, and integrity. Recognizing and accepting claims on this is what we are calling "reasoning from principles."

And there is a practical problem about debates framed in terms of conflicts among rights, a problem that the abortion controversy also illustrates: The rhetoric of rights escalates the intensity of feelings and

hardens positions, reducing any opportunity for compromise or for taking adequate account of new information. Feelings, while human and
important to recognize, are not an adequate basis for resolving conflicts
of values, as we have already discussed in this chapter. People who
insist on talking in terms of rights—rather than what would be good,
fair, or just, or even the best outcome in a situation—have often passed
well beyond the point at which they may be receptive to compromise or
other ideas. For this reason, even if we had a better understanding of
what rights are and who has what rights, attempting to resolve ethical
issues by appealing to rights could have a powerful, counterproductive
effect.

We know that people have legal rights. Do people also have moral
rights? The answer to both questions is yes, people have both legal
and moral rights. But these rights are not the same. And while both
are important, all we are saying at this point is that trying to resolve
ethical problems by framing those problems in terms of conflicts
among rights is generally an unproductive strategy. In general, we
suggest that when people frame issues in terms of conflicts among
rights, one way to move the discussion in a more productive direction
is to try to get people to talk about which are the most important values that they are trying to express and why those values are seen as
being so important. Considerable tact and sensitivity are often
required to accomplish this, but can often lead to a willingness to
approach issues from a perspective more open to mutual understanding and, sometimes, compromise.

FOLLOW YOUR CODE OF ETHICS

One response within the health professions to the erosion of public confidence has been to develop and promulgate codes of ethics. This
response is not new. In fact, the medical branch of the health professions
still prides itself on the tradition associated with its earliest code of
ethics, the Hippocratic oath, even though fewer new physicians now
actually swear it. That oath runs as follows:

> I swear by Apollo Physician and Asclepias and Hygieia and Panaceia and
> all the gods and goddesses, making them my witnesses, that I will fulfill
> according to my ability and judgment this oath and covenant: to hold him
> who has taught me this art as equal to my parents and to live my life in
> partnership with him, and if he is in need of money to give him a share
> of mine, and to regard his offspring as equal to my brothers in male lin-
> eage and to teach them this art, if they desire to learn it, without fee and

covenant; to give a share of precepts and oral instruction and all other learning to my sons and to the sons of him who has instructed me and to pupils who have signed the covenant and have taken an oath according to the medical law, but to no one else.

I will apply dietetic measures for the benefit of the sick according to my ability and judgment; I will keep them from harm and injustice.

I will neither give a deadly drug to anybody if asked for it, nor will I make a suggestion to this effect. Similarly I will not give to a woman an abortive remedy. In purity and holiness I will guard my life and my art.

I will not use the knife, not even on sufferers from the stone, but will withdraw in favor of such men as are engaged in this work.

Whatever houses I may visit, I will come for the benefit of the sick, remaining free of all intentional injustice, of all mischief, and in particular of sexual relations with both female and male persons, be they free or slaves.

What I may see or hear in the course of the treatment or even outside of the treatment in regard to the life of men, which on no account one must spread abroad, I will keep to myself holding such things shameful to be spoken about.

If I fulfill this oath and do not violate it, may it be granted me to enjoy life and art, being honored with fame among all men for all time to come; if I transgress it and swear falsely, may the opposite of all this be my lot. (Temkin and Temkin, 1967)

Now, how does the Hippocratic oath bear on current ethical problems? Consider this case:

Case 2.8: Hippocratic Oath as Code of Ethics

Dr. Gregory P. argues against assisted suicide on the grounds that he, "like all physicians, is bound by the Hippocratic oath." Dr. Jack K., on the other hand, points out that even though the oath prohibits physicians from giving "a deadly drug to anybody if asked for it," Dr. P. prescribes such toxic drugs many times a day. "Besides," laughs Dr. K., "I don't suppose you 'will not use the knife, not even on sufferers from stone' or teach medicine without a fee. And really, Gregory, do you still sacrifice a cock to Apollo Physician, Asclepias, Hygieia, and Panaceia before attending to patients?"

Of course, Dr. K. is being overly literal in his interpretation of the Hippocratic oath, making the point that Dr. P.'s use of this oath to justify his stance against assisted suicide is only one way to read the oath and what it stands for. But this is an important point: not only ancient, traditional codes, but also contemporary ones require interpretation, and differing interpretations are still sometimes consistent with what the codes actually say. Thus, one problem with substituting professional codes of ethics for ethical decision making is that codes are somewhat ambiguous guides to behavior. Even when they do address pertinent issues, codes require interpretation.

Of course, no code can address all the ethical issues practitioners are likely to encounter over a career. And uncritical acceptance of any code of ethics is an evasion of personal responsibility, for accepting a code of ethics as one's own guide to behavior is a moral, not a technical, or a practice, decision. But even if one accepts a code in good faith, no code of ethics is an adequate substitute for capable moral reasoning because of problems inherent in codes themselves.

Let's look at one example of these problems: codes express values without indicating how they are to be applied. For instance, the American Nurses' Association (ANA) Code for Nurses says, among other things, that "The nurse participates in the profession's efforts to establish and maintain conditions of employment conducive to high quality nursing care." But does this mean a nurse is unethical if she continues to work for an employer who reduces staffing to a dangerously low level? Or would she be unethical if she abandoned those patients by resigning? After all, the ANA code also says that "The nurse acts to safeguard the client and the public when health care and safety are affected by the incompetent, unethical, or illegal practice of any person" (cited in Benjamin and Curtis, 1992, p. 220).

The conflict between these two elements of one code illustrates another problem of codes of ethics: internal inconsistency. But even when codes provide helpful guidance, choices dictated by codes still require justification to nonadherents (people who are not members of one's own profession). And, unfortunately, many ethical issues do involve people, such as colleagues in other health care disciplines, who do not share the same code and who, therefore, may not regard the code of someone else's profession to be valid, let alone binding on them. When the values of different codes conflict, they can actually contribute to counterproductive, interdisciplinary squabbles. Additionally, one may be conscientiously opposed to provisions of the code. And, as portions of the Hippocratic oath make clear, codes may become antiquated through moral progress and new information.

Finally, the consensus-developing process by which codes become professionally accepted often leads to excessive reliance on platitudes, concerns about malpractice law, and avoidance of controversial issues. So codes often fail to give guidance when it is most needed. This is not to say that codes are worthless; they can and do express the consensus values of professions and set a kind of minimal standard of practice. But for all the reasons stated, they are not equivalent to fully responsible ethical decision making.

FOLLOW PROFESSIONAL PRACTICES

The last unsatisfactory substitute for fluent ethical reasoning that we will discuss here is in some ways the most familiar of all. It is to model one's own behavior on the practices of others in one's profession. After all, each of the health professions requires or imposes a period of mentorship and apprenticeship, as well as a period of probation, on those entering into practice. And what one learns during those mentoring and probationary periods is not merely technical; it also concerns attitudes, standard operating procedures, and, most importantly, values. Can we responsibly accept the behavior of others in our profession as a guide to ethical decision making?

Case 2.9: Problems with Local Standard of Practice

Community Hospital has two surrogate consent/permission forms. One requires that a competent patient assign responsibility to a substitute in case the competent patient is unable to make decisions at some later time; the other, a moribund patient form, assigns responsibility usually to next of kin, when the patient is incapable of informed consent. In reviewing charts, Dr. Charlie S., an intern, is surprised to find moribund patient forms transferring responsibility to family members, only to visit the patients and find the patients alert and apparently competent. In the locker room, other doctors tell him not to worry about this discrepancy, since it's so time-consuming to explain everything to patients and get them to sign all the consent documents. "There's never been a problem," Charlie is told.

The decision to model one's concept of ethical practice on the consensus of practice is itself a moral decision that requires justification both to oneself and to others because it is based on the assumption that the behavior of others is itself morally defensible. But, after all, there is good reason for Charlie to doubt that the consensus of practice regarding consent forms at Community Hospital is ethically acceptable. So, more generally, before one models one's behavior on that of others, one would need to judge their behavior to be ethically responsible in advance of imitating it. In fact, to be confident that copying the consensus of practice will produce ethical results in one's own situation, one would also have to know that the situations in which others have made their decisions are relevantly similar to one's own, that no new information has come up that would affect the decision, and that no preferable options are available. We must also recall, as mentioned earlier in the chapter, that the interpretation of professional roles, and therefore the modeling of them, is ambiguous, unclear, and not a firm basis for ethical decision making. Thinking through all these questions is ethical reasoning, in which case "consensus of practice" is not really a substitute or even a shortcut. Perhaps more important, such a reliance also delays moral progress and the improvement of professional standards because it uncritically accepts the "going rate" as acceptable, even when it isn't.

Moreover, because the standards current in a profession are not self-evidently justified for those who are not members of that profession, those outside of one's profession will still require a justification in terms of values they share. For example, if financial managers tend, as a group, to disregard others' interests in their concern over financial values, it does not follow that their insensitivity will be regarded as ethically tolerable by those whose interests are ignored. For all these reasons, modeling behavior on that of others in the profession without carefully thinking about the standards of practice and ethical behavior they may or may not be living up to is not fully ethically responsible.

Now, it is very important to think carefully about what we have explored in the last two chapters. In effect, we have found good reasons to question what are certainly the most common approaches to "ethical" decision making in health care and, for that matter, in American society more generally. The temptation will be strong to accept these criticisms on a superficial level, but not actually take them to heart in ways that will affect our own decision making. This temptation will be particularly strong because we have not yet offered a positive alternative (that is the project of the next several chapters of this book). But, again, thinking back on all the ideas of this chapter should give us good reason to be receptive to a more satisfactory alternative than any of the approaches considered here. The task now becomes the identification of at least one alternative that is clearly more satisfactory from a professional ethical point of view.

QUESTIONS FOR DISCUSSION

1. A number of explicitly religious groups are currently active on the American political scene, attempting to influence public policy in directions consistent with their ethical views. Examples of some issues of concern to the Christian Coalition are promoting prayer

in public schools, securing government financial support for private religious schools, and opposing abortion. Some other religious groups, however, including a number of Christian organizations, have opposed the Coalition's involvement in these efforts to influence public policy. Granted that all parties to these issues have a right to freely express their ideas in an attempt to influence public debate, does (should) a religious affiliation strengthen or weaken their influence? In a society that both protects religious freedom and separates church (synagogue, temple, mosque) from state, what should be the role of religious belief in public policy debates with ethical dimensions?

2. Most hospitals and many other health care institutions post a Patients' Bill of Rights statement. Examine the Patients' Bill of Rights posted in any institution with which you have some connection. Are you surprised by any of the rights listed there? Are all of those rights routinely respected? How would you determine whether or not your institution is in compliance with its rights statement? Are the rights listed sufficient to assure patients that they will always receive respectful, dignified treatment? Why or why not?

3. The American Nurses' Association Interpretive Statement 1.1 of the ANA Code of Ethics (1985/1994) includes the following passage:

> The fundamental principle of nursing practice is respect for the inherent dignity and worth of every client. Nurses are morally obligated to respect human existence and the individuality of all persons who are the recipients of nursing actions. Nurses therefore must take all reasonable means to protect and preserve human life when there is hope of recovery or reasonable hope of benefit from livesaving treatment.

How would this portion of the code apply to Rosa's case? Remember, she's asking for required disclosure of HIV status from patients, especially those who might be homosexual. How would this portion of the code provide guidance for the dilemma concerning treatment of Jonathan, whose father opposes transfusion on religious grounds? In *Ethics in Nursing,* Benjamin and Curtis (1992) observe that

> To respect the "dignity" and "individuality" of the client [in their example] seems to require that his autonomous refusal be honored. But to "preserve human life when there is hope of recovery or reasonable hope of benefit from lifesaving treatment" seems to require that his refusal be overridden. Which should it be? (p. 9)

4. *Case 2.10: Religious Beliefs and Professional Practice*—James is a substance abuse counselor in a state-funded program who often uses a twelve-step approach modeled on Alcoholics Anonymous. A deeply committed evangelical Christian, James firmly believes that placing oneself in the hands of a higher power is an indispensable step in recovering from substance abuse. He welcomes the opportunity presented by this step in the program to witness to his own faith and encourage his clients to accept Jesus into their lives as well. Are there any ethical issues involved in this situation? How should situations like this be handled?

CHAPTER THREE

An Approach to Ethical Decision Making

AN ETHICAL DECISION PROCESS

Having discussed some of the most common substitutes for ethical reasoning, we now need to offer something to put in their place. While the content of this chapter is far from a full-scale ethical theory, we offer it as a provisional guide to ethical decision making—provisional in the sense that we will not try to justify it in terms of traditional philosophical argument. Instead, pending fuller discussion of ethical theories in later chapters, we offer this approach as a practical guide to ethical decision making. We will apply it to two ethical problems, one in the context of individual practice and the other in the context of an institutional ethics committee.

Case 3.1: Dilemma Concerning Confidentiality

For some time now, Jamie P. has been concerned about her friend and fellow occupational therapist, Candy R. Over a period of months, Candy has become increasingly moody and withdrawn, working with her clients with an attitude of barely controlled impatience and even hostility, though not, so far as Jamie knows, actually abusing or neglecting them. Gathering her courage, Jamie finally decided to talk with Candy about her concerns; Candy proposed stopping at The Fern Bar after work.

Much to Jamie's surprise, Candy was well aware of her problems and explained that she was currently working her way out of a cocaine problem she had developed over the past year or so. She was not, she said, making use of their employer's substance abuse program because the promise of confidentiality was routinely violated: "It would be all over the place in no time." Besides, Candy said, she was "handling it OK on my own." She attributed the behavior Jamie was concerned about to the effects of withdrawal and expressed confidence, now that she had been drug-free for over a month, that her problems would subside. In any event, Candy insisted, Jamie was not to tell anyone, certainly not their supervisor. What should Jamie do?

Jamie's ethical dilemma is, unfortunately, all too common, and it is an extremely stressful one. On the one hand, Jamie would naturally feel some loyalty to Candy. Candy's confiding in Jamie also creates a kind of obligation: presumably Candy would not have said anything if she had felt Jamie might pass it on. Moreover, Jamie and Candy are colleagues; one consequence of violating Candy's trust will certainly be a poisoned working relationship. On the other hand, Candy's behavior has been sufficiently problematic that Jamie's concern for Candy's clients was aroused. Jamie has a clear professional obligation to assure that Candy's clients' interests are not affected by Candy's problems. And, presumably, Jamie would feel some concern about Candy's own situation. People with substance abuse problems are not always truthful, especially about their ability to "handle it OK" on their own. How, then, should Jamie make a professionally responsible, ethical decision in this case?

Step 1: Problem Identification   First, Jamie needs to gather, understand, and represent accurately all the facts that are relevant. This step is absolutely crucial in all ethical decision making, even though there will almost always be information one would want but is impossible to get or impossible to get without violating other important values. In this instance, it would certainly be important to investigate Candy's work carefully to determine whether or to what extent her problems have interfered with her effectiveness as an occupational therapist. It would also be important to determine that Candy has actually overcome her substance abuse problem and is now drug-free. Candy herself might or might not be cooperative in providing information like this, and Jamie will need to think carefully about how to gather and verify it without alienating Candy. But without this kind of information, Jamie cannot make a responsible ethical decision.

It is also extremely important that Jamie stick to the facts, rather than allowing assumptions and suppositions to masquerade as legitimate information. For example, although it may be true that people with substance abuse problems are often untruthful, it would not follow from this, or any of the facts of this case as presented, that Candy is being untruthful or indeed that she still has a substance abuse problem. What certainly is factual, even without further investigation, is that her professional behavior was erratic and troubling enough that Jamie became concerned by it. But Jamie should be careful about drawing unjustified conclusions from her behavior alone.

> *What do you think are the most important facts Jamie needs to find out? How should she go about getting the facts she needs?*

Step 2: Values Identification   Jamie should now identify all of the values at stake in this situation and decide on an approximate priority order of these values. To some extent, she has already done so: one cannot have an ethical problem unless one has at least some sense of what values are coming into apparent conflict. Trying to identify these values specifically, however, is a necessary step in resolving the issue. In this case, there are values concerning Candy's professional conduct; her physical and emotional well-being; her trust and confidence in Jamie; her desire for respect, privacy, and confidentiality. There are also values concerning Jamie's professional responsibilities, her concern for Candy and her concern for their clients, her obligation to her employer and her supervisor. There are values concerning all those who have been or might be affected by Candy and Jamie's practice and behavior. Which of these values should be considered the most important may be difficult to decide, though in cases of this kind client welfare would normally be extremely important.

> *What do you think are the most important values involved in this situation? (Be thorough!) Which of these values would you rank as more important? Which are less important? (Remember, Candy is at least a colleague and maybe even a friend. Put yourself into this situation.)*

Step 3: Option Identification   Jamie should consider all her options. At this point, evaluating her options can get in the way of brainstorming them, so she should restrict herself to thinking up possibilities. She has a number of them. She could do nothing and maintain confidentiality. She could do nothing right now, but monitor the situation, intervening later if the occasion warrants it. She could report Candy's conversation with her to her supervisor and/or the substance abuse counselor. She could maintain confidentiality about their conversation, but report her observations concerning Candy's practice problems to her supervisor. She could inform Candy of her intentions or conceal them from Candy.

Step 4: Consequence Identification   Jamie should now identify the relevant possible consequences of each option and which values will be promoted or sacrificed by each possible choice. Of course, it may turn out that some options violate Jamie's highest-priority values and will therefore be eliminated from consideration very quickly. But it is often useful to think through all the consequences as a way to open a sufficiently broad range of possibilities.

Doing nothing and maintaining confidentiality would preserve many loyalty and working-relationship values, as well as meeting many of Candy's concerns, but it does little or nothing to safeguard client welfare and may risk allowing unprofessional conduct. Monitoring the situation enhances information, contributes to respecting Candy's values, and, to some extent, helps safeguard clients. But it places a heavy burden of responsibility on Jamie, who, of course, has other demanding obligations of her own. It also implicitly undermines their supervisor and their employer's efforts to deal effectively with substance abuse issues.

Reporting the conversation to a supervisor and/or the substance abuse counselor supports them in their responsibilities while lifting the burden from Jamie. It also safeguards clients and may contribute to Candy's eventual rehabilitation. But it destroys Candy's trust; alienates her from Jamie; wrecks their working relationship; and, if Candy is right about the substance abuse program's lack of confidentiality, exposes Candy to professional ruin. Reporting her concerns but not their conversation respects Candy's desire for confidentiality as well as the obligations and responsibilities of their supervisor and contributes to safeguarding clients. It also has the great merit of not going beyond the facts—that Candy's work behavior has been a cause of concern. Informing Candy of Jamie's intention treats Candy honestly and respects her autonomy, but may provoke angry feelings of meddling and loss of trust. Not informing her can be construed as dishonest and manipulative but, at least temporarily, preserves a more amicable working situation.

Step 5: Option Selection   Jamie should choose that option which sacrifices the fewest high-priority values and yields the best balance of good consequences. In this situation, we suggest Jamie ought to report her concerns about Candy's work to their supervisor (but not the substance abuse counselor), yet maintain confidentiality about their private conversation and carefully refrain from speculating about the cause of Candy's apparent problems. We also suggest that Jamie ought to tell Candy that this is her intention. While Candy may be unhappy that Jamie intends to pursue the matter at all, they both presumably share the deep value of client well-being as a primary obligation; and even in this case Candy may come to see that Jamie is behaving with scrupulous professionalism by sticking strictly to the facts that may be relevant to the value of client welfare. But even if Candy does not recognize this, she is being treated respectfully as well as compassionately by Jamie if she follows this course of action.

Did you come out with the same resolution we did? There is room for disagreement, depending on how you ranked your values and what other options you may have thought of. Remember, the goal is not to get universal consensus. It is to get a responsible resolution that sacrifices as few high-priority values as possible.

Step 6: Documentation   Finally, a narrative of how Jamie arrived at her decision—that is, how she worked her way through steps 1 through 5—provides an explanation and justification of her decision that is likely to be acceptable to any but the most emotionally involved parties. That is, we think it is not naive to hope that Candy will perhaps eventually come to understand the ethical responsibility exhibited by Jamie's resolution of the problem. And we also think that other parties, such as institutional superiors and clients, will also accept her judgment as ethically responsible. But the acceptance of her judgment will crucially depend on the thoroughness with which Jamie has worked through each of the steps. If, for example, she has overlooked one or more worthwhile options or has ignored or underestimated values important to any of the parties, they are unlikely to accept her narrative as a justification of her decision.

Reminder: the six steps in ethical decision making are

1. *Problem identification: all the relevant facts surrounding the dilemma. The who, where, and what?*

2. *Values identification: identification and prioritization of all the values at stake. The why?*

3. *Option identification: all the possible solutions to the dilemma. What are the options?*

4. *Consequence identification: the result of each option. What if we do . . . ?*

5. *Option selection: sacrificing the fewest high-priority values. What's the best choice?*

6. *Documentation: summarizing each step as well as the conclusion in a narrative.*

ETHICAL REASONING IN GROUPS

Of course, not all ethical issues arise in such a way that there is only one decision maker. Ethical issues often affect more than one person: departments, entire institutions, or even communities, regions, or society as a whole can be involved. So it is not uncommon, especially in the highly institutionalized setting of contemporary health care, to find that ethical decisions wind up being negotiated by groups.

Among such groups with special responsibility for ethical decision making are what are sometimes called institutional ethics committees (IECs). The rise of IECs in American hospitals and long-term-care facilities is a comparatively recent phenomenon. But many accreditation

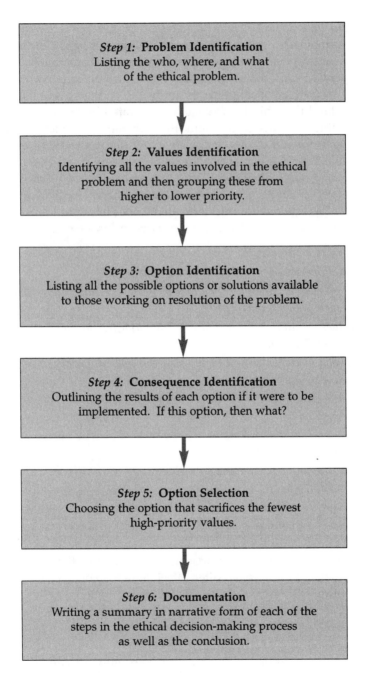

Figure 3.1   *Ethical decision-making process.*

agencies now require them, though efforts at monitoring and promoting their effective use still have a long way to go. As discussed earlier, several historical issues have been especially influential in propelling the development of IECs. One is the ruling of the New Jersey Supreme Court in 1976 that Karen Ann Quinlan's father could legitimately direct that her ventilator be turned off and other support withdrawn, together with the suggestion that further such cases could be resolved by hospital ethics committees (Pence, 1990).

Still another influential factor is the dramatic escalation of malpractice suits, together with the fear that this escalation inspires among health care practitioners. Groups as diverse as the President's Commission for the Study of Ethical Problems in Medicine, the American Medical Association, and the American Hospital Association have all supported the role of ethics committees in resolving patient care dilemmas at the hospital, rather than turning to the courts (Bayley and Cranford, 1986). It is important to remember that the decisions of IECs are not normally considered legally binding. However, the recommendations of IECs, especially when cogently reasoned, have generally been respected by the courts.

In spite of these factors, there has been considerable resistance to the establishment of IECs, as well as great reluctance to assign them a meaningful role in institutional decision making. Some health care providers feel threatened by what they perceive as a judicial body potentially unsympathetic to their actions, composed of members with varying, sometimes negligible clinical expertise and uncertain loyalties. Physicians may feel that "IECs threaten to undermine the traditional doctor-patient relationship and to impose new and untested administrative and regulatory burdens on patients, families, and physicians. Their existence may shift the focus of decision making from the office or bedside to the conference room or executive suite" (Bayley & Cranford, 1986). Hospital administrators are understandably reluctant to have incidents involving questionable practices brought to a committee that may include people not directly affiliated with the hospital. Neither are they eager to have internal management decisions subjected to additional scrutiny. And there is also a potential for conflict of interest between the IEC's responsibilities to individual patients, as well as colleagues and staff, and the efforts to minimize hospital risk, develop sound policies, and allocate resources.

As we shall see, most of these concerns are ill-founded, at least when an IEC is properly set up and operating effectively. And, at most institutions, health care providers have found that, as IECs have matured, their advantages greatly outweigh any disadvantages they might have been thought to have. Health care providers are often most anxious about bringing patient care issues to institutional review boards or ethics committees because they fear that they may be criticized or blamed, or even disciplined. The focus of effective ethics committees, however, should be on recommending improvements in approaches and policies, rather than on judging individuals or offering advice on clinical issues. In order to avoid some of these anxieties and promote a broader conception of the role of institutional ethics committees, we will apply the six-step guide to ethical decision making offered for case 3.1 to an example that does not address patient care.

Case 3.2: Dilemma Concerning Conflict of Interest

National Hospital Supply's Laser Technology Division is offering to fund travel and accommodation expenses for the laser safety officer, chief of internal medicine, and chief of surgical staff to attend a one-week seminar in Hawaii on the advantages and proper uses of its new products. (The actual seminar amounts to two three-hour sessions.) National has a reputation as the Mercedes-Benz of equipment: excellent quality, but costly. All three staff members sit on the budget committee that will recommend equipment priorities for the upcoming budget cycle. The director of purchasing would like a recommendation from the ethics committee concerning what she feels may be a conflict of interest.

Many features of this case make it quite different from Jamie's dilemma. For example, the ethical dilemma in the National Hospital Supply case is far more difficult to identify and understand. However, the first step—to gather, understand, and accurately represent all the relevant facts—remains the best way to start.

Some clarification would be in order. The committee is responding to a request from the director of purchasing, but it is not clear what kind of recommendation is being asked for. (These kinds of ambiguities are common in IEC requests.) At a very early stage, then, the committee should clarify this matter. And probably it will turn out that the director is not merely looking to the IEC for confirmation of her sense that there may be some conflict of interest in this case. Probably she is asking for guidance about whether or not to ask the hospital staff invited by National to refuse or cancel their trip. And, given the way that institutions typically work, she may be asking for something even more far-reaching: a policy recommendation about permissible and impermissible inducements or benefits donated by vendors.

Step 1: Problem Investigation   Assuming that the committee is invited to deal with these broader issues, it would be important to determine exactly what National Hospital Supply's proposal is, as well as how the affected staff understand it. On its face, the proposal bears some suspicious features: Hawaii is a famously desirable and quite expensive tourist destination; the seminar lasts an entire week, of which only six hours is actually spent learning about new products. So, in effect, the staff members are receiving what appears to be a free six-day vacation trip, all expenses paid. While the clinical areas of the invited staff do bear a reasonable relationship to the products being demonstrated, it is likely that other staff members who are not on the budget committee would have equal or better abilities to evaluate the merits of National's products. So, one might suspect, this offer could be an attempt to exert undue influence on future purchase decisions. The purchasing director's concern about conflict of interest amounts to the fact that the staff may feel a conflict between (1) their obligations to the institution to determine equipment priorities on such bases as frequency of use, serious need, and cost effectiveness, and (2) appreciation for National's hospitality.

It is important to note that such an apparent conflict of interest need not reflect ethical discredit on the staff involved. They may be quite capable of preserving their objectivity about equipment purchases, and their motives may be irreproachable. However, this situation does lend itself to suspicion. And whether that suspicion turns out to be deserved or not, suspicion itself is a fact that must be taken into consideration.

Some additional facts may be relevant: Virtually all hospitals have policies prohibiting staff from accepting gratuities (tips). Businesses are legally prevented from paying bribes and kickbacks, though not from maintaining good customer relations. Many purchasing departments seek to limit vendor access to other staff. However, gray areas abound. For example, it is not at all unusual for vendors to pass out small gifts, such as coffee cups and pens with company logos on them, or to bring pizza or a meat-and-cheese plate to a department lounge. Fruit baskets are common at Christmas, and various kinds of contributions to staff parties are not unusual. But such "freebies" are not evenly distributed in hospitals; the bulk go to departments, like surgery, with large budgets and extensive equipment needs.

Step 2: Values Identification   The committee must identify all the values at stake in the situation and decide an approximate priority. Clearly, the hospital has a strong interest in making its budgeting decisions objectively, unencumbered by any competing loyalties, as well as in promoting an atmosphere of confidence in its decisions. More generally, the hospital has an interest in holding down expenses, and these expenses are increased not only by buying costly equipment, but also by the expenses that vendors incur for their "freebies." But the hospital also has an interest in the continuing education of its staff, as well as in their morale; allowing vendors to provide seminars and "freebies" contributes to these ends. And the invited staff members clearly have educational and recreational interests in accepting National's proposal.

This situation is further complicated when considerations of fairness, treating similar cases similarly, enter in. Staff members who are not the recipients of favors from vendors often resent the fact that other departments seem better treated. And institutions do not always have much control over vendors. Many recipients of vendor proposals are not hospital employees and so cannot be compelled to follow policies that are binding on staff. But this distinction carries little weight among staff: if Dr. X brings a vendor to a department meeting, it is both awkward and disruptive to try to prevent him from speaking; however, it sets a precedent that bringing in vendors is generally acceptable. Besides, most professional organizations of health providers have not taken the lead in reducing gray-area vendor contributions: many appear to encourage lavish spending by suppliers at national conventions, for example.

The values of institutional integrity are clearly very important and outweigh individual or collective staff desires. The interests of vendors in having fair access to potential buyers and of buyers in having fair access to ethical suppliers are clearly important too, but the key term here is "fair" access; what National appears to want is something more—a sense of indebtedness, or personal access to decision makers. Accordingly, that value should not receive a high priority; it conflicts directly with much more important values, such as fairness, as well as important institutional priorities.

Step 3: Option Identification   Next, all the options must be considered. One option, of course, would be to limit the IEC's response to the narrow issue of whether there may be a conflict of interest in this case and not make a recommendation concerning whether the staff should be permitted to accept National's offer, leaving that decision to the chief operating officer. Another option would be to make a recommendation concerning this particular offer, but not to make a general policy recommendation, leaving such matters for case-by-case consideration. In this case, one option would be to recommend permitting the trip; another would be to recommend against it; a third might be to recommend that those going on the trip not be members of the decision-making budget committee; and a fourth might be negotiating a different, less costly way for National (and its competitors) to educate the staff concerning their products. Another option would be to attempt to formulate a general policy concerning vendor offers. Such a policy might be to permit all donations that are not unlawful and allow vendors to decide for themselves what they want to do. Another option would be to attempt to discriminate permissible from impermissible vendor contributions, perhaps by placing a dollar limit or restricting the kinds of items that may be donated. Or the IEC might seek to recommend banning all such contributions.

Step 4: Consequence Identification   Identifying all relevant possible consequences of each option and which values will be promoted or sacrificed by each one is the next step. Even though the IEC's decision will be a recommendation (since IECs do not have enforcement powers), relevant consequences should include the effects of putting any recommendation into general practice, as well as the fact that any policy will have limited application and enforcement (for example, because not all physicians involved are hospital employees). Concerning the first option, unless it is very clear that the director of finance is really only interested in having her diagnosis confirmed, the IEC will probably appear to be evading its proper role by legalistic hairsplitting. Besides, the chief operating officer is ultimately responsible anyway, so this option does nothing special to promote values of institutional integrity.

Case-by-case evaluation has the merit of enabling fine distinctions to be made, but it creates the impression of potential unfairness and consumes an immense amount of institutional time and energy. Offering a recommendation on this particular case without any broader policy recommendation also creates the appearance of arbitrariness, while establishing potentially problematic precedents. Perhaps, then, a recommendation on the National case should follow from a policy decision.

Among the policy options, leaving the issue up to vendors risks grave abuses; the integrity of the hospital's decision-making processes would be impaired, and suspicions and charges of unfairness and favoritism would be rampant. A strict prohibition has the merit of simplicity and would, if followed, help restore confidence and potentially reduce costs. But it would be unenforceable, promote hypocrisy and deviousness, and undermine morale. Setting some sort of limit risks arbitrariness and brings with it its own problems with enforcement, but at least reduces the seriousness of potential conflicts of interest. At the same time, it is realistic; it is, in effect, what most honorable vendors do.

Step 5: Option Selection   Now the option that sacrifices the fewest high-priority values and yields the best balance of good consequences must be selected. We think it is likely that a policy limiting vendor contributions probably achieves this. Spelling out the exact terms of the limits is necessary, but difficult; perhaps the permissibility of "freebies" might be a judgment call by the director of purchasing, based on moderate cost and "innocence." A policy based on this recommendation might require all vendors on hospital grounds to be wearing a badge issued by the director of purchasing before contacting any hospital staff. Badges would be issued contingent on vendor agreement to honor the hospital's limitations on access and contributions.

But now, what follows from this recommendation concerning National's offer? We think the trip should be (politely) refused on the grounds that it is unreasonably expensive and suspicious. We also think that the director of purchasing ought to negotiate with National (and other suppliers) to provide less lavish opportunities for staff to become acquainted with their products, so that objective, well-informed decisions can be made concerning equipment.

Step 6: Documentation   Finally, we think this policy should be aggressively promoted among all staff, including those associated with, but not employed by, the hospital. Our justification and written documentation would cite all the considerations above in steps 1 through 5.

MORE ABOUT ETHICS COMMITTEES

In the preceding discussion, we applied the guidelines for ethical decision making to a case involving an institutional ethics committee. However, we did not discuss the composition or membership of the IEC, nor did we explain its working in any detail. One reason for these apparent omissions is that the composition and membership of IECs varies greatly, as do their internal workings. Regrettably, many IECs are constituted in ways that do not reflect much institutional confidence, and they often make many of the mistakes we discussed earlier in terms of individuals. That is, some IECs are designated as a home for kindly, well-intentioned, but not especially influential staff members. Other IECs are staffed as if ethical decisions were essentially practice problems, financial issues, labor negotiations, or religious or legal issues. While all these perspectives and values can be important, we stress that unless the IEC includes members with significant training in ethics, the committee will function well only by accident.

Several types of dysfunctional IECs are fairly common. *Nominal ethics committees* exist on paper, to satisfy accreditation requirements, meeting perhaps once or twice a year, affirming platitudes about ethics, but doing no real work. *Fig leaf ethics committees* exist to find ethical justifications for decisions based entirely on financial considerations, institutional efficiencies, or risk reduction. *Debating society ethics committees* see themselves as forums for discussion of interesting cases, but nothing more. In debating societies, everyone is supposed to present concerns and perspectives, no matter how relevant or (un)informed, but venting is the only result, not policy or other recommendations. *Tribunals* see themselves as charged with reviewing staff decisions retrospectively for the purpose of approving or disapproving and acquitting or chastising the decision makers. Such IECs usually put themselves rapidly out of business by alienating everyone they are supposed to serve.

So what are institutional ethics committees for? According to the President's Commission, effective IECs "have emphasized their consultative, advisory, informational, and consensus development roles rather than primary decision making" (President's Commission, 1984). Effective IECs can play valuable roles in (1) providing counsel and support to health providers and to patients and families, (2) offering opportunities to discuss and recommend options and alternatives in cases with significant ethical tensions, (3) assisting in resolving issues concerning life support and extraordinary means, (4) recommending institutional policies that facilitate patient-centered care and responsible practice, (5) promoting institutional arrangements that are adequately sensitive to ethical considerations, and (6) fostering an environment of ethical awareness. They should not, of course, make patient care decisions in place of responsible care providers, either directly or by the quasi-authority of the group, though they can and should suggest options. They should not provide the opportunity for health care professionals or administrators to abdicate their proper responsibilities. And they should not allow themselves to become nominal, fig leaf, debating society, or tribunal ethics committees.

TYPICAL SOURCES OF CONFUSION
IN THE PRACTICE OF ETHICS

The examples of ethical decision making we have just considered have been drawn from actual practice, but they were somewhat simplified in order to illustrate the approach to ethical reasoning presented in this chapter. In real life, matters are almost always more complicated. In closing, we want to identify a number of these complicating factors as a kind of warning about what one can expect outside the classroom.

First, it is often difficult to give moral values a sufficiently high priority in ethical decision making within an institutional context. So far, we have not discussed moral values as distinct from other values in any detail; instead, we have only insisted that ethical decision making involves identifying all the values at stake in the situation and deciding on an approximate priority among them. Values like fairness and justice, trust and confidence, and the like have guided our discussion, but further explanation must wait until the chapters in Part II on ethical theory.

Nevertheless, it is often difficult to avoid pressures to substitute legal, economic, or institutional decisions and decision-making processes for moral ones. Most health care delivery in America is inextricably bound up with complex institutions: hospitals, insurance companies, government oversight agencies, and the like. These institutions are composed of people with varying interests and perspectives, some of which can come into conflict with ethical decision making. While most health care providers are morally sincere people, it is natural that other concerns may seem to them more important than what someone else may consider ethical. Thus, for hospital risk managers and legal counsel, no course of action that exposes the provider to legal risk will appear justifiable, no matter how morally compelling the arguments may be for it. To the finance department, if ethical considerations seem to require an imprudent cost, so much the worse for ethical considerations (or, to put the matter more sympathetically, it is unlikely that finance would find imprudent expenses to be ethical). Union contracts or administrative considerations may sometimes require practices that, on consideration, are ethically dubious (for example, making staff assignments based on seniority alone or requiring managers to honor personal days off regardless of low staffing or risks to patients); yet considerations of institutional convenience may make it difficult or impossible to modify these questionable procedures.

In practice, then, it is often difficult to avoid substitution of legal, economic, or institutional priorities for actual ethical decision making. Legal, economic, and institutional values are important and they can seem less abstract than other values common to ethical dilemmas. As ethically responsible health care professionals, this fact increases our responsibility to keep ethical decision making sensitive to a broad range of values besides these familiar ones.

A second obstacle to ethical decision making related to the institutional structure of health care delivery involves the tendency of institutions to engage in hierarchical diffusion of responsibility, bureaucracy, and evasion. "Hierarchical diffusion of responsibility" refers to the fact that institutions are often set up in such a way that it is difficult to identify any particular individual who is accountable for any particular questionable action or decision. Responsibility is often referred to persons higher up in the organization, but farther and farther removed from actual practice, and therefore less and less directly responsible. Moreover, there often appear to be no consequences for such persons once they do accept responsibility. When the vice president of a hospital says, "I take full responsibility for the actions of my staff," those words can be an entirely empty gesture if no actual changes result. And such meaningless actions undeniably undermine efforts to practice ethical health care. To those affected, such behavior appears to be nothing more than an evasion of ethical responsibilities by burying them in bureaucracy.

A third related point is that people on the front lines of health care face difficult, highly stressful day-to-day experiences. Most naturally turn to their colleagues and coworkers for support. But ethical issues can prove divisive, undermining confidence and mutuality in working relationships. Moreover, ethical criticism often prompts retaliation, while a more positive response is usually dependent on the very goodwill that may be destroyed by the criticism. Under these circumstances, it is easy to understand that people may be reluctant to speak out on ethically questionable practices or behaviors. It is common to turn a blind eye, to "judge not lest ye be judged," to avoid "throwing stones." It is common to evade responsibility by pretending that unwillingness to speak out is really tolerance of differing values or to pass the issue up the hierarchy of institutional authority, where, all too frequently, the issue is likely to get shoved under the rug, because "it's not up to me." Thus the need to preserve good working relationships can lead to disregard of ethical priorities.

A fourth kind of problem arises when people lack confidence that ethical issues can really be resolved at all. "Everyone has different values" has become such a platitude that the great extent to which people actually share basic values can get lost, and with it the hope that reasoned agreement can be reached. A few high-profile issues contribute to this sense that ethical issues are intractable: the abortion controversy, euthanasia, and physician-assisted suicide. But, as we shall see in the next chapter, the ethical theory that underlies this anxiety is very dubious. And, as we have already seen, it is possible, and sometimes even easy, to think our way through ethical dilemmas to widely, if not universally, acceptable solutions. Ethical decisions can be easier to achieve when ethical decision making is viewed as a deliberative, participatory process. It also gets much easier with practice.

Now we come back to a point made earlier. There are, we observed, essentially two kinds of ethical issues, the normative (knowing what is the right thing to do) and the motivational (doing the right thing once one knows what it is). The four considerations discussed here are essentially motivational, though they are sometimes brought into the normative debate in order to cloud that fact. Hard as it may be to achieve, ethical practice requires a courageous combination of integrity, sympathy, and tact. It also requires the patience to work steadily to heighten the responsiveness of health care institutions to ethical values, even when those values may be inconvenient. Economic, legal, and institutional priorities have many advocates; they are seldom far from the center of concern for risk managers, administrators, and others. It is therefore critical that those who provide health care articulate and defend ethical values and decision making, taking the responsibility not only to practice ethically, but also to advocate the interests of patients, clients, and society generally.

QUESTIONS FOR DISCUSSION

1. Think of an ethical problem you are familiar with. Then apply the problem-solving procedure discussed in this chapter to that problem. How does it work?

2. What, exactly, is wrong with bribes, kickbacks, gratuities, cash-back promotions, vendor-paid parties, "freebies," and the like? Or, if they are not all ethically suspect, where should the line be drawn and why there? If you were the director of purchasing in case 3.2, what would your criterion for permissible and impermissible vendor "freebies" be? Why?

3. *Case 3.3: Suspicion of Family Abuse*—Keesha R. is a home-care nurse visiting Mrs. Pi, who is occasionally lucid, but mostly confused. She is also subject to violent mood swings, sometimes lashing out at people or objects around her and sometimes injuring herself. Her primary caregiver is her son Paul, who is outspokenly resentful of the problems his mother presents, but who has also been reasonably conscientious in the past.

    On this visit, Mrs. Pi's face is bruised, and she is acting uncharacteristically timid; she appears afraid and actually cowers when Paul, who smells like alcohol, is in the room. In response to Keesha's questions, Mrs. Pi denies that there is anything wrong. But Paul chimes in that "there damn well might be if people don't start minding their own business and leaving them alone." Following the procedure given in this chapter, determine what you think Keesha ought to do in this situation.

4. Do any of the hospitals, clinics, nursing homes, or other health care institutions you are involved with or know about have institutional ethics committees? If so, have you or anyone you know ever taken an ethical problem to the committee for its consideration? If so, how well did it meet your needs? What might have been done to meet them more successfully? If not, why not? What would it take to get you to submit an ethical issue to an IEC?

PART II

An Introduction to Ethical Theory

In the next three chapters, we explore the most common moral or ethical theories actually held by people in contemporary society. Ethical theories are patterns of reasoning about apparent conflicts among values and normally include a background analysis of what ethical values are as well as a procedure for figuring out what is the most ethically responsible thing to do in a problematic situation. One reason we study ethical theories is to help us diagnose correctly the ethical reasoning patterns of those around us, including our own, so we can understand them better. Another reason to study ethical theories is to be able to anticipate likely problems associated with one or another approach to ethical reasoning as well as any strengths they may have. A third reason to study these theories is that with understanding, we can be more effective in articulating value issues and working toward responsible resolutions.

As in the earlier chapters of this book, we examine some unproductive patterns of ethical reasoning—because even though these patterns are not professionally responsible, they are regrettably common. So we need to know how to respond when people approach ethical issues in these unproductive ways. But we also discuss more productive and responsible patterns of ethical reasoning. These will supplement the approach to ethical decision making we offered in Chapter 3.

With regret, we must report that we cannot offer a single, unambiguous, universally acceptable ethical theory, much less a simple ethical recipe to resolve ethical problems. We will ultimately suggest that there are three approaches—reasoning from principles, reasoning from consequences, and reasoning from character (or from virtue, including some feminist perspectives on the matter)—each of which has considerable validity and each of which may have a legitimate role to play in the resolution and justification of ethical decision making. Often these approaches converge; sometimes they do not. A thorough understanding of the strengths and weaknesses of each can assist us in determining how best to make use of their strengths and avoid their weaknesses in actual ethical decision making.

CHAPTER FOUR

Egoism and Relativism

RELATIVISM

Relativism is the traditional term for theories that share the idea that there are no objective, interpersonally valid ethical values. This idea can take many forms, however, and we cannot examine all of them. Instead, we will look at several of the most common. We begin with a relativistic theory called *egoism* that focuses on the individual in a very special way.

Case 4.1: The Selfish Surgeon

Dr. Guevara is one of the most technically proficient cardiovascular surgeons on the staff. He is also one of the most difficult human beings patients and staff have ever had to deal with. Before every difficult case (and most of the rest as well), Dr. Guevara becomes enraged at delays, equipment problems, illnesses among "his" team (which he insists on personally selecting; he has been known to call in people who were on vacation and pull people from other cases). He then rants at and abuses anyone in earshot. His equipment requests are often three to four times more expensive than those of other surgeons, and he is utterly unreceptive to any suggestion that priorities other than his are also important. Finally, Dr. Guevara is extremely territorial: he takes very aggressive (and sometimes underhanded) measures to prevent any other physician from "horning in on my practice."

Dr. Guevara's reasoning is relativist in the sense that he does not acknowledge the interpersonal validity of any values. For him, the only values that count at all are his own interests. This position is often called *ethical egoism*. Egoists reason as if an action's ethical value or "rightness" consists in its tendency to advance their own interests. Sometimes, egoists like Dr. Guevara are simply blind to the interests of others (*naive egoism*). Sometimes, but not always, egoists extend the same reasoning to others and hold that actions right for someone else are actions that

59

advance their interests (*universal egoism*). And, sometimes, egoists hold that although others may have interests important to them, everyone else ought to sacrifice their interests so that the egoist himself is better off (*individual egoism*).[1]

In spite of its repellant selfishness, egoism has a number of features that seem attractive to some people. First, egoism seems consistent with the widespread idea that human beings are basically self-interested agents and with the related idea that the basic point of society is to allow people to satisfy their interests to the greatest extent possible (or to the greatest extent compatible with a similar opportunity for others). Second, egoism seems consistent with the idea that if people would simply mind their own business and look after their own interests, everyone would be better off. Third, if ethical behavior just boils down to self-interested behavior, getting people to do the right thing will be less of a problem; it's simply a matter of getting them to see how the right thing is in their self-interest. And, fourth, if ethical egoism is true, there is less difficulty figuring out what is the right thing to do; one simply determines what is in one's own interest and does that. In short, egoism offers a simple solution to both the motivational and the normative problems in ethics.[2]

However, these apparent advantages do not stand up to careful consideration. First, the idea that human beings are basically self-interested (egocentric) does not entail that they always act only in their own self-interest or that, when they do, they behave ethically. In fact, it seems likely that most people do, at least sometimes, act in self-sacrificing, or altruistic, ways: think of donating blood, for example, or the more heroic sacrifices people make for loved ones or more abstract causes. Moreover, it also seems likely that when people act self-interestedly, they sometimes act very unethically indeed, which is why "selfishness" is generally regarded as a moral failing. This lack of ethics should be especially clear in the cases of naive egoism and individual egoism. People who run

---

[1] These distinctions among types of egoism, as well as many of the criticisms that follow, are developed from material in Brian Medlin's "Ultimate Principles and Ethical Egoism," *Australasian Journal of Philosophy*, 35 (1957).

[2] Although egoism has lacked persuasive philosophical advocates, it has not lacked spokespersons. Perhaps the most famous and accessible is the novelist and "objectivist" Ayn Rand, whose rich ideas of self-interest and rationality are often unfairly caricatured. The tradition of caricaturing egoists is very old; Plato, for example, does it to Callicles in the *Gorgias* and to Thrasymachus in the *Republic*, where, however, Plato tries to provide a detailed refutation of the position. It is important to remember that scoring at the expense of egoists is not at all the same thing as showing in what ways they are wrong.

roughshod over the interests of everyone else, either through ignorance or through self-centeredness are not behaving ethically; they are merely selfish. Since they make no effort to address apparent conflicts of values, their behavior cannot be considered ethical at all.

Second, it is simply not true that if people would mind their own business and look after their own interests without regard for others, then everyone would be better off. Some important human interests can be satisfied only at the expense of others, so that those whose interests are sacrificed will not be better off if the strong and successful look after only themselves. Some people are simply much less able to look after their interests than others: children, for example, as well as the elderly, the disabled, and many others. Moreover, some important human interests require self-sacrificing cooperation for success (most team or group activities do, for example). So, if everyone seeks only to maximize his or her own interests, these activities either would not be accomplished or would cause a good deal of resentment on the part of those carrying the self-interested "free rider."

Some further explanation of the problem may be in order. Some human interests, such as team- or group-based activities, require self-sacrificing cooperation to achieve desired outcomes. When egoists are involved in a group activity, they may reason that their interests are best served by appearing to cooperate with the group while, in fact, doing as little as they must and only if it benefits them directly, and by allowing (or compelling) others to do whatever requires any sacrifice of hard work, time, energy, and the like. The egoist thus takes advantage of the group's efforts, while the group has to work harder to carry the egoist, who is getting, in effect, a "free ride." Groups normally resent such behavior bitterly, and egoists who are not highly skillful manipulators often suffer various forms of retaliation.

But consider the problem from the egoist's point of view for a moment. To be consistent with the principles of egoism—that right actions are the ones that benefit the self—the egoist would have to encourage others to sacrifice their interests for his or hers. After all, to encourage others to look after their own interests would reduce the egoist's chances of taking unfair advantage of them. So, it appears, egoism requires a kind of hypocrisy: deceptive and manipulative pursuit of self-interest for oneself, the promotion of self-sacrifice for others. In reality, such a frame of mind is probably too conspiratorial for most egoists, who are probably only naive, simply paying no attention to the consequences of their self-centeredness on others, rather than cynically manipulating them. That there is an implicit hypocrisy in egoism, however, is hard to miss once it is pointed out.

In light of these observations, it seems pointless to claim that egoism solves the problems of knowing the right thing to do, as well as being motivated to do it. If, as should be obvious, there are situations that call for self-sacrifice, the temptation to ignore one's responsibilities cannot be an unambiguous guide to ethical behavior. However, there is another problem with the way egoists make ethical decisions that deserves attention. Notice that egoism provides an especially unpersuasive rationale for ethical judgments. As we have seen, people will normally regard any decision as unjust unless it is clear to them that their interests have been given fair weight in the decision-making process. But, by definition, the egoist does not take the interests of others into account; the judgments of egoists reflect nothing more than their best guess about their own interests. Not surprisingly, then, other people affected by them almost always feel that egoists' decisions are unethical. And for that reason, among others, egoism is not a professionally defensible approach to ethical decision making.

Now, it may seem that we are spending too much time on an approach to ethics that is self-evidently inadequate for any responsible professional. Unfortunately, egoists are not as uncommon as this feeling suggests. What, then, should we do when we encounter someone like Dr. Guevara? Though it may be difficult to remember this at the right time, if human beings are not just cynical self-interest maximizers, and they are not, our attitudes toward each other can and should become a little more charitable. Excessive concern for oneself is a moral failing. But since people are also capable of compassion, disinterested altruism and kindness, generosity, love, and a wealth of other, unself-interested feelings and motives, we can and should hope that even the most embittered and cynical egoist can possibly be reached. On this analysis, Dr. Guevara, and egoists more generally, are morally underdeveloped, and we ought to do what we can to educate them.

At the same time, it is important to remember that egoism has at least one valid point to make. It would be unrealistic to ignore the importance of self-interested motivations in getting people to do the right thing once they know what it is. When people are hesitant to do the right thing, it is often because the apparent cost in terms of sacrificing their own interests is simply too great. When this conflict occurs, it becomes indispensable to show them that, however long the run and uncertain the result, ethical behavior really does "pay off" in some sense important to them and their interests. In some cases, however, making this point successfully can be very difficult, and it is always possible that there may really be no direct payoff compelling enough to persuade the one whose sacrifice appears morally necessary. Thus, the motivational problem in ethics is very serious indeed; we must not underestimate it.

> *Not all persons share the same ideas of what values are important. Individual value preferences are based on life experiences, personality, culture, ethnicity, religion/spirituality, and more. Our global community is, after all, pluralistic. However, ethical reasoning can result in a convergence of values that many can and do accept.*

Some students may feel that the biggest problem with egoism is not so much the central role it gives individuals in deciding their own interests and acting on them, but its unreasonably narrow conception of the interests people normally choose. Most people just aren't as self-centered as egoism suggests. People do sometimes focus only on their own desires. But it is more normal for people to act on a whole range of interests and values, many of which will include promoting the interests of others whom they care about. Parents do, after all, sacrifice their interests for their children; friends promote each other's interests; and many people make huge sacrifices for their churches, civic organizations, and countries. But not everybody shares the same ideas of what values are the most important. And certainly different people work to promote differing values in many differing ways. So it seems true that the causes and people that individuals value are up to them; we all, as people say, have different values. And to many people it seems arrogantly intrusive, as well as unreasonable, to attempt to judge someone else's values as better or worse, more or less right or good, than some other set of values.

This set of considerations contributes to an ethical theory that differs from egoism by recognizing the complexity of individual values without abandoning the idea that ethical values are fundamentally individual commitments. The next case shows what such a theory might look like in practice.

Case 4.2: Agree to Disagree?

Dr. Kawabata's willingness to take on virtually any surgical procedure under virtually all circumstances has earned him the nickname "the Samurai Surgeon." Recently, several of his cases have provoked considerable concern among his colleagues, as well as the nursing staff. Their concerns were of two kinds: it appeared to some that Dr. Kawabata took on cases he was not really well-qualified for and "muddled" or "improvised" his way through them, thus jeopardizing patient welfare. And it appeared to others that Dr. Kawabata performed procedures, especially on terminal patients, from which no significant benefits could reasonably be expected. When called to discuss these issues with the practice council, Dr. Kawabata pointed out that "It's up to each individual to make his or her own judgments about what is and what is not ethical practice. It might seem to others that some of my judgments were questionable, but then I probably think some of their judgments are questionable. Who's to say who's right? People have to make up their own minds."

In this case, Dr. Kawabata's argument is that of an *individual ethical relativist*. Individual relativists believe that no action is simply right or wrong all by itself; instead, what someone considers ethical depends on his or her beliefs and feelings. So an action may be morally right for one person and wrong for other people, depending on what values each person accepts as binding on him or her. So, if pushed by the practice council to explain his actions further, Dr. Kawabata might point out that others' criticisms are really only a matter of differing perspectives. Every professional performs cases for the first time, after all; if no one undertook cases he was not already experienced doing, no one would ever become competent in any new procedures. Besides, whether or not a patient will benefit from a treatment is essentially a judgment call each professional has to make personally. It might even be irresponsible to base such judgments on some impersonal standard-of-care criteria that don't leave room for individual differences.

We want to emphasize that Dr. Kawabata and individual relativists generally are usually completely sincere in their emphasis on the importance of individual differences concerning values and actions. After all, relativism does offer some very attractive features. First, each individual's responsibility to develop sincere, personal values and act on them is taken very seriously by this theory. Second, it highlights and explains the obvious truth that people do differ over values: different people, different perspectives, different life experiences, and different feelings will obviously produce different values. Third, it emphasizes the importance of tolerance, a virtue that is increasingly valuable in a pluralistic world and that contributes greatly to an effective working environment by diffusing confrontations.

Yet most of us would probably be uncomfortable with the implication that Dr. Kawabata's relativistic ethics render him immune to any form of professional review. Certainly it is not characteristic of contemporary health care practice to reject the validity of review by one's peers on the grounds that their values apply only to them. And there are other problems with individual relativism. If our values are up to us, not only is there no obvious basis for any form of moral or ethical education, but all forms of ethical judgment of others also lack justification. So it would be hard to reconcile individual relativism with efforts of the professions to develop codes of ethics and hold their members to high standards of conduct. And, lastly, justifying our own decisions to others by citing individually relative feelings and commitments is likely to be exactly as unsuccessful as citing only egoist considerations. If our values are up to us, why should patients or superiors care about Dr. Kawabata's?

Societal Relativism

What seems wrong about individual relativism, at least to many people, is that it does not sufficiently emphasize the fact that certain kinds of groups recognize that certain ethical norms are binding on members of the group and that it is the right and responsibility of group members to articulate, encourage, and expect compliance with those norms. Some of these are societal standards or expectations; others may derive from professional or other roles and affiliations. And differing societies or groups certainly can and do articulate, encourage, and enforce compliance with different norms. But, at least within the framework of group values, ethical conduct can be understood as conduct consistent with accepted norms. This idea is also compatible with the value of individual freedom as regards lifestyle choices, personal loyalties, and differing interests, at least in relatively free societies.

A traditional designation for theories of this kind emphasizes the social role in developing values by calling it *societal relativism*. A societal relativist believes that an action's ethical standing depends on its being consistent with the norms (values, beliefs, feelings) held by most members of the society to which the agent belongs. Thus, an action may be right for an agent who belongs to one society and wrong for an agent who belongs to a different society. Extending this societal relativism idea further, ethically responsible actions for any member of a group or profession within society will depend on the values shared by members of that group or profession. So, for example, the standards of truthfulness expected of criminal defense lawyers may be different from the standards of truthfulness considered professionally ethical by loan officers.

Societal relativism solves some problems with other forms of relativism. For example, it provides a clear and convincing basis for moral education: every society initiates its own members into its values, as do many groups with distinctive value commitments. And it does address the binding force of ethical judgments among individuals who participate in the same framework of values. At a somewhat deeper level, it does seem that virtually all imaginable valuation rests on some community of evaluators who share similar criteria for judging, which is consistent with societal relativism's emphasis on group valuation. And it does seem to explain some changes in values over time: as society changes, its values similarly develop. So, for example, as American society has become less tolerant of racism, some of racism's more overt forms, such as legal segregation, have become morally intolerable.

Societal relativism does, however, leave a number of troubling issues without convincing resolutions. For example, it undermines the validity of any intersocietal moral judgments, as when one nation accuses another of violating basic human rights. And, of course, the members of one society would have no reason to accept as binding on them the judgment of any other society. So a racist society could perfectly well reject criticism on the grounds that the ethical standards involved are those of the critic, not of the racist society. But this line of thought flies directly in the face of the idea that there are basic and universal human rights. And it also conflicts with the idea associated with the Nuremberg trials, that even if one engages in grossly inhumane conduct because one is following the lawful orders of one's superior (or society), one is still ethically responsible.

> *Unfortunately, societal relativism does not serve as a bridge between groups. Moral behavior expected of one group may not be congruent with the values, beliefs, and feelings of another group. But, in health care, as in life more generally, we often have to work with a diverse collection of people who feel allegiances to many groups and many competing values. What we need is a pattern of ethical decision making that will enable us to resolve situations of this kind.*

Here is another interesting point. The history of human culture includes a number of great moral leaders and ethical teachers. Probably most people would include Mohandas Gandhi and Martin Luther King, Jr., among that number. Notice, however, that neither of these moral leaders advocated or practiced the societal status quo; both, in different ways, rejected the dominant values in their societies. Moreover, it was the fact that they did call those dominant values into question that made them moral leaders. But, if societal relativism is right, it would follow that, to the extent they violated dominant values, Gandhi and King were not great leaders and teachers, but rather thoroughly unethical wrongdoers who deserved, at the least, severe moral censure. And the point can be generalized beyond the level of whole societies. For example, if it is common practice to misrepresent a used car's actual qualities to conceal its defects, it would follow that an honest salesperson would be unethical if he told the truth.

So the fact that a society or group within society shares certain values does not justify or validate those values for anyone who might question them, either within or outside of that society. The fact that some societies endorse gross violations of human rights does not make those violations ethically defensible.

Finally, here are four general observations about relativism from the standpoint of professional ethics. First, relativism fails to guide behavior in morally problematic situations—because what normally makes a situation ethically problematic is that, as individuals or as members of society, we have no clear ethical values to guide our actions. (For example, if we ourselves are unsure what we think about physician-assisted suicide, then—given the deep split among members of society generally—how can relativism help us resolve our ethical uncertainty?) Second, relativism provides no persuasive justification for moral judgments to assist professionals in defending moral choices. Not only are individual and societal values not universally accepted, but it's also pretty clear that, at least in some cases, they shouldn't be. Third, as we saw in Dr. Kawabata's case, relativism may rule out professional peer and self-review by denying validity to any criteria other than those one accepts for oneself. And, fourth, societal values may conflict with the values of other groups to which we belong; how, then, do we decide which set of values takes priority and what justifies our decision? Unless there is some set of values or some set of procedures with a validity greater than individual or group commitment, these questions will probably remain unanswered.

Even though there is some validity to egoism, individual relativism, and societal relativism, none offers a satisfactory approach to professional ethics (Table 4.1). Egoism fails because it does not address ethical problems as ethical—as situations in which apparently conflicting interests need to be accommodated on terms that assign relevantly similar interests relevantly similar weight. Relativism of either kind is a genuine problem because it can become a near insurmountable obstacle to resolving any interpersonal ethical dilemma; the parties to the discussion give up reasoning with each other and "agree to disagree" on the grounds that what is true for you is true for you and what is true for me is true for me. In a sense, relativists simply demand that people take moral intuitions at face value, without any further justification than the fact that somebody feels a certain way or that such and such is accepted by this or that society.

Relativists and egoists are attempting to confront serious issues: the fact of ethical disagreement, the fact that individuals need to accept responsibility for their own ethical values, the fact that societies and other groups have profound influences on which values people accept,

Table 4.1   *Forms of Egoism and Relativism*

Concept	Definition	Comments
Egoism	Ethics based on advancing interests of individual person.	Behavior is based purely on self-interest without regard for how behavior may affect others.
Naive egoism	A form of ethical unawareness of the interests of others.	Individual is unable to recognize the legitimate interests of others.
Universal egoism	Each individual pursues his or her own self-interest, and encourages others to do so as well.	Individual recognizes that others have legitimate interests, but does not acknowledge any responsibility to further others' interests.
Individual relativism	Ethics based on values, beliefs, and feelings of one individual for him- or herself.	The interests of others are recognized but deemed relevant only for those who share those interests.
Societal relativism	Ethics based on the values, beliefs, and feelings of a group to which the individual belongs.	Consensus values of groups are deemed normative for individual members of those groups.

and the fact that people are often motivated by self-interested considerations. However, it is important to see that the solutions proposed by relativists and egoists involve a number of serious mistakes.

While it is true that individuals differ on some important moral issues, it is also true that they agree on far more than they disagree on. The moral universe is the same for everyone in that it is based on concern for human dignity, decency, voluntary relations that are not oppressive, and some kind of spiritual fulfillment. These norms, which make up moral lives, are construed differently at different times, in different places; and the particulars vary depending on our capabilities (we are all similar, but we're not identical), the evolution of local histories and customs, and the models generated for their expression. But the basis of concern is the same. Despite the differences in human values reflected by differing traditions and priorities, we need to work and act together in ways that respect core ethical concerns. Thus, it is important that moral ideas are validated by ethical reasoning to ensure that these ideas have the interpersonal authority to guide responsible practice.

Therefore it is reasonable to say that while people hold conflicting values, their high-priority values are remarkably uniform. And this uniformity of core concerns is what offers the best chance that patient, sympathetic reasoning can lead to resolutions in situations of ethical conflict.

It is probably true that most people acquire their moral ideas from the process of socialization they experience in their particular society and that most people do pass through a series of developmental stages in their ethical thinking. But it does not follow from this that the moral ideas people are socialized into are therefore morally right or that the changes in their moral ideas are necessarily progress—that is, movement toward morally better ethical understanding. This is one mistake many philosophers associate with the social sciences: the tendency to pretend that their supposed "descriptions" are somehow value-free or objective when in fact they operate on concealed value judgments. The process by which people acquire ideas is not the same as the process by which those ideas are proved to be sound. And moral ideas need to be proved to be sound if they are to have any rational claims to interpersonal authority.

This, finally, is the crux of the problem of relativism for professional ethics. As long as the only justification of one's decisions is relative to the decision maker or decision-making body, it is hard to see why anybody else has any reason to accept it as valid for them as well. The inescapable arbitrariness and irrationalism of relativism makes it an unsatisfactory basis for professional ethical decision making or practice.

QUESTIONS FOR DISCUSSION

1. *Case 4.3: Hustling Clients*—Every fall, Dr. Browne, a counseling psychologist in private practice, offers a free lecture to the Parent Teacher Association at her children's school on learning problems and psychological therapies. In addition to the public education she provides, she hopes to receive more referrals from these parents. Do you think her behavior is professionally ethical? Why or why not?

2. If relativism is not valid and there are at least some interpersonally valid ethical standards, why is tolerance or respect for autonomy important? Why not just identify the interpersonally valid standards and get people to live up to them?

3. *Case 4.4: Consciousness Raising*—Anita is an outspokenly conservative, antifeminist colleague in the lab. She believes and urges others to believe that women are properly subordinate to men and that women do not deserve equal pay for equal work;

she opposes the union ("We're all just lucky to have a job; we have no business making demands") and is the sole support of her unemployed husband, whom she serves in every possible way. Would it be improper to try to talk her out of some of these beliefs? Is there any kind of ethical responsibility to try to change her mind? Why or why not?

4. Are there actually deep differences among core ethical concerns? Or do you agree that "while people hold conflicting values, their core ethical concerns are remarkably uniform"? Give examples from your own experience that tend to support your view of this question.

A COMBINED THEORY

After reading the previous section you might be impatient with the discussion of egoism and relativism that appears there. People who consider the matter carefully may suspect that the forms of egoism and relativism we have presented do not really represent their underlying validity very well. Instead, it may seem that we have constructed versions of these theories that are especially vulnerable to criticism. So, in this section, we want to try to capture what may well be the most common ethical position actually lived out by conscientious people in contemporary American society.

First, we suspect very few health professionals present themselves as egoistically as Dr. Guevara, or as relativistically as Dr. Kawabata, at least in the workplace and provided that they have an opportunity to think about their position before having to represent themselves to others. Most health professionals recognize that daily practice involves constant compromises and accommodations of competing interests, and most also recognize that those compromises and accommodations need to be at least reasonably fair. At the same time, the conflicting demands made on professionals in practice make it nearly impossible to afford the luxury of being a disinterested, rational observer. Everyone involved in health care is constantly placed in a position of arguing aggressively and competitively for his or her own interests, those of his or her patients or clients, those of his or her department, and the like. There are never enough resources to meet every legitimate need. Accordingly, an excessive sensitivity to the interests of others might actually interfere with fulfilling one's obligations to one's own patients and colleagues.

Second, health care, like society generally, is becoming more diverse, both in terms of levels and kinds of training and in terms of perspectives and values practitioners bring to the workplace. While there may be a convergence of standards for clinical practice among disciplines and specialties, tolerance of individual and group differences concerning values is an essential ingredient in an effectively functioning health care system.

Third, on top of demanding and difficult work situations, many health care providers are also people whose lives are buffeted by immense social and personal problems. Many statistics demonstrate that people in health care are especially prone to divorce, alcoholism, drug use, and many other more socially acceptable indicators of excessive stress. Realistically, then, it may be fruitless to expect that health care professionals will be able to live out lives that reflect nothing but adherence to the highest, most unyielding ethical standards, whatever those are.

Perhaps the most realistic idea about ethics would be to try to live up to the highest practical standards of professional conduct in one's role as a health professional and recognize the immense diversity of values and coping strategies people live out in their private lives, as long as no one else is seriously affected for the worse. That is, perhaps the most reasonable health care ethic would be one that combined a rigorous professional ethics at the workplace with a general commitment that people ought to be free to live out their own, individual values outside the workplace, provided that those values do not harm others. Let us call this a "combined theory" because it puts together elements of a role-based, principled professional ethic with a relativistic private morality, limited by an absolute prohibition against harming others.

What would such an ethic be like? At its best, it might well lead people to be responsible professionals, as well as self-actualizing individuals both sensitive to others' needs and tolerant of differences concerning values and interests. However, consider the following case.

Case 4.5: Combined Theory—Who's to Judge Private Acts?

The affair between Dr. Cheney and Liz Jackson, one of the hospital pharmacists, was a hot rumor in the locker rooms and over the lunch tables, but the gossip was especially uncomfortable for Anna R., one of Jackson's colleagues in the pharmacy, because Dr. Cheney's wife, Carole, is Anna's cousin and lifelong friend and because Anna's husband plays on the same softball team as Liz's husband. One afternoon, Anna, who had not seen Liz for a while, unlocked the door to the break room and found Cheney and Jackson embarrassedly breaking off a sexual encounter.

Both urged Anna not to tell anyone, especially not their spouses. "What we're doing doesn't hurt anyone," they said, "and we're not going to break up our marriages over this. But we're in love; we can't help it. Telling Carole would only hurt her, and telling Bob would crush him emotionally. And, anyway, it's really none of your business what we do, as long as we do our jobs and nobody gets hurt. Who are you to judge, anyway?"

In this example, Cheney and Jackson are not merely egoists or relativists. They are acting on the combination of ideas described above: professionalism in their workplace roles, following their personal feelings (values) in private, and observing the need not to harm others. More specifically, Cheney and Jackson are implicitly claiming three things. First, so long as their actions do not negatively affect their workplace functioning—so long as their affair is conducted "on their own time"—no colleague has any ethical obligation or grounds for complaint. Underlying this point is that both Cheney and Jackson do accept a responsibility to maintain appropriate standards of professional functioning in their workplace roles ("as long as we do our jobs").

Second, they are implicitly claiming that their personal relationship, being separate from their professional relationship to each other and others, is a matter of private morality and therefore not an appropriate subject for ethical evaluation by a colleague. That is, while Cheney and Jackson might accept that Anna could have a legitimate basis for complaint if their affair constituted some kind of professional malpractice, as long as they meet all their professional responsibilities competently, Anna has no legitimate basis for judging them negatively. However, third, they are implicitly acknowledging that others ought not to be harmed by their actions and are inviting Anna to share that judgment by urging her to withhold any disclosure of their affair.

Let us begin by considering each of these claims separately. Although both Cheney and Jackson do accept the idea that they have professional ethical responsibilities, it is not clear exactly how they know what these are. It is most likely that they are equating role-based responsibilities with ethical responsibility. As we have already seen, however, such an equation cannot be considered an adequate professional ethic. Among other reasons, role-based ethics is an evasion of responsibilities that may transcend any particular role. If Cheney and Jackson are thinking of their professional responsibilities merely in terms of clinical adequacy alone, their view of professional ethics is too narrow and self-serving.

To put the point less abstractly, Cheney, Jackson, and all other health care professionals have an obligation not merely to diagnose and provide therapy and dispense accurately, but also to be people in whom others can confidently place their trust, on whose judgment they can rely, and who are, at a minimum, honest and sincere in their dealings with others. Clearly, however, their affair undermines all of these expectations, and others besides, because conducting an affair requires deception and the violation of trust at the most fundamental level possible. To the extent that they engage in this affair, then (and not even counting the extent that others, like Anna, are put in compromising positions by their affair), Cheney and Jackson are already violating their professional responsibilities and attempting to coerce others to do so as well. What they do "on their own time" does unavoidably affect their work because it makes them into the kinds of people who cannot live up to the legitimate professional expectations of others. Being a true professional is more than doing your job competently. It is being the sort of person who lives up to demanding and honorable standards of personal behavior in public and private. Here again is a point we've made several times: your private life affects your professional life, and vice versa. To pretend otherwise is dishonest as well as unprofessional.

Then consider the claim that personal behavior apart from professional relationships is not an appropriate subject for ethical evaluation. There is certainly something appealing about this idea. Most people would be uncomfortable without at least some privacy in their lives, where they can do what they want without feeling that they are on display or that their actions are subject to review by others. This feeling is especially strong when it can be coupled with the idea that harming others is the boundary beyond which such private behavior is no longer immune to criticism.

However, it is obvious that some private actions are legitimate causes of concern. Actions that seriously harm the people who engage in them—including at least some kinds of recreational drug use—are among these. Even the most outspoken civil libertarians usually acknowledge a moral responsibility to intervene when someone constitutes a "clear and present danger" to himself or herself, though one does not wish to be too paternalistic in defining the danger. Of course, religious authorities have always emphasized the spiritual harm that entirely private but immoral actions can produce. But one need not be religious to agree that certain kinds of pornography, for example, can erode someone's sensitivities in profoundly troubling ways.

But beyond the potential for harm of one kind or another, it seems plausible that there are some actions that are intrinsically wrong, quite apart from whether or not they harm others or those who engage in them. In Cheney and Jackson's case, it seems plausible that their dishonesty and violations of trust are wrong whether or not their spouses— or anybody else—ever find out about them. So it is not at all obvious that not harming others is a sufficient criterion for ethical conduct.

Cheney and Jackson are also making a claim that not harming others not only justifies them in deception and dishonesty, but also constitutes sufficient reason for others—Anna, in this case—to engage in deception and dishonesty as well. There is a real question whether the spouses of Cheney and Jackson might not be better off in the long run knowing about the affair and confronting it directly; if that is the case, their being told about the affair might not ultimately be a harm. This does not mean that Anna herself has an obligation to inform their spouses; that is clearly a much more debatable issue. Still, discovery cannot but be painful for all the parties in the short run. Does that fact oblige Anna to lie?

We do not think so. If Anna gives in to Cheney and Jackson, she will help to contribute to an environment in which deception, disrespect for people, and lack of self-control are all acceptable norms. She will also, in effect, give up the right and responsibility to make her own moral decisions, rendering herself captive to others' unethical behavior; her own integrity, trustworthiness, and decency are lost if she joins the conspiracy. It is, after all, Cheney and Jackson's affair that puts others in harm's way. Trying to make Anna responsible because of her discovery—to make her seem like a nosy, interfering, prudish busybody—is only another dishonest evasion by Cheney and Jackson.

There is an important general point to be made about this "no public harm/leave us alone" ethic and morality. It fundamentally ignores the fact that, in addition to being individuals, we are all parts of a larger human community (many communities, actually) toward which we owe obligations of decency, civility, trustworthiness, and genuineness. All too often, people confuse a legitimate expectation of individual liberty with an extreme, isolationist individualism, according to which we are all only narrow self-interest maximizers in ruthless competition with every other isolated individual. But society—human community—is more than an arena in which isolated individuals struggle to get desired goods for themselves. Society is a complicated network of mutual activity in the service of health, education, art, music, literature, worship, and so on performed by people who share a deep commitment to important values beyond their own immediate gratification. Indeed, it has been argued that unless people have such a genuine, mutual commitment to values beyond their own happiness, that happiness can never come.[3] Since such mutual activity and commitment requires confidence that can be destroyed by many kinds of seemingly private actions, those actions cannot be ethically neutral.

As professionals, as people, we have ethical responsibilities beyond competence, self-gratification, and not harming others. We have, among others, responsibilities to foster confidence and trust. This does not mean we ought to become moral vigilantes or fanatics. But tolerance, taken too far, can amount to negligence, ignoring one's responsibilities to educate people morally or to get involved in other ways. And this, in turn, can lead to the radical erosion of the quality of life—to a constant stream of indignities and dissatisfactions of daily existence, a sense of meaninglessness, and the sense of living in an unfeeling, uncaring, fragmented, and inhumane world. Such an ethic is clearly unsatisfactory.

We are now in a position to see much more clearly why we do not attempt to draw a sharp distinction between professional ethics and private morality. First, trying to draw such a distinction ignores the many ways one's own character (personal life) affects one's professional life. The kinds of people we are inevitably transcend any artificial professional boundary. Our values, professional and personal, make us who we are and contribute to our sense of self-respect. Second, it requires a kind of ethical schizophrenia to adopt one set of values at home and another in one's profession. We think, on the contrary, that the kinds of values that make people moral also make them ethical: honesty, integrity, competence, compassion, and so on. Third, we deny that all private morality ought to be immune from ethical evaluation. We think some behavior consistent with certain values may just be intrinsically wrong, regardless of who is helped.

QUESTIONS FOR DISCUSSION

1. How and why, if at all, would your thinking about case 4.5 change if

   a. Cheney and Jackson were both pharmacists? Both were groundskeepers?

   b. Cheney is unmarried and Jackson is separated from her husband pending a divorce?

---

[3] This is because happiness is a by-product of doing things that are actually worth doing. But unless we care about the things we do, and not just the happiness we want from them, we will never get the happiness we hope for. Doing things we don't care about cannot produce happiness. A persuasive presentation of this argument can be found in Joel Feinberg's "Psychological Egoism," published in *Reason and Responsibility*, ed. Joel Feinberg (Encino, Calif.: Dickenson, 1965).

c. Cheney and Jackson were never openly affectionate at the workplace; Anna accidentally interrupted their tryst at a staff party given at another surgeon's house?

d. Jackson is Cheney's boss?

2. *Case 4.6: Romance with a Former Client*—John is an occupational therapy student intern at an inpatient mental health facility. There he strikes up a friendship with Brenda, a patient, though she is not his client. Two weeks after Brenda's discharge, John calls her; they begin to date. Six weeks later, however, while they are still seeing each other regularly, Brenda readmits herself to the facility. Does John have any professional obligations concerning this new situation? What should he do? Why? How and why, if at all, would your thinking change if

a. John and Brenda had dated prior to Brenda's first admission?

b. Brenda had called John and initiated the social relationship after her initial discharge?

c. Brenda's readmission is related to John's unwillingness to allow the relationship to develop due to ethical concerns about the circumstances under which they met?

d. John has requested reassignment to a different facility; Brenda, however, has herself referred to that facility because she wants to "keep in touch with" John?

3. Do you agree that some actions are simply wrong regardless of whether anyone (or anyone besides the agent) is hurt or harmed by them? What are some of these? (Be specific; you might draw examples from your own experience.) What makes them wrong?

4. *Case 4.7: Private Versus Professional Conduct*—Bearing in mind that one may not have a responsibility to "blow the whistle" on unethical behavior in every case, which of the following do you think raise serious professional ethical questions or concerns? Why those and not the others? What, if anything, should you do about each case? Paula is a member of your staff who

a. runs the smoking cessation program but, off-site, smokes two packs a day.

b. has embezzled funds at your church; the board has decided not to publicize or prosecute, since Paula seems genuinely sorry and has agreed to return the money.

c. has soft-core pornography discreetly mailed to her at work to conceal this interest from her husband and children.

d. houses (or employs) illegal aliens at home.

CHAPTER FIVE

Consequentialism and Ethical Principles

CONSEQUENTIALISM

Case 5.1: Which Floor to Close?

Low occupancy rates in several units of Community Hospital make it necessary to close at least one floor indefinitely. Studies done by staff to generate the relevant information indicate that most of the functions and staff from the orthopedic unit can be spread to surgical or pediatric floors but not vice versa. Which of these floors would be the best choice to close?

All other things being equal, it would seem reasonable to close the orthopedic unit because the fewest people would be affected and the greatest diversity of services would be preserved. This decision was reached by means of a pattern of reasoning called "consequentialism," which involves choosing as ethically the best option the one that will probably maximize good and minimize bad results. The net balance of good and bad results is sometimes called an option's *utility*. Familiar under other names, such as "cost-benefit analysis," consequentialism is a natural and common method of decision making in health care and other fields. The value recognized is utility and its broad application. Consequentialism is also a goal-driven pattern of reasoning. One particular form of consequentialism, called *utilitarianism*, is certainly among the ethical theories most widely defended by philosophers, though it also has influential critics. In this chapter we examine consequentialism and ultimately recommend that, when suitably circumscribed, consequentialism can be a defensible approach to professional ethical decision making.

A general definition of consequentialism might run as follows: a decision is morally right (ethical) if the sum of its results is at least as good as any alternative decision that might have been made in the same circumstances. But this definition is still compatible with many alternative forms of ethical reasoning. And, unless we are careful to specify that the "sum of its results" means all the effects of a decision on all those whose interests are affected, this form of consequentialism can be compatible with some unethical patterns of reasoning as well: egoism, for example, maximizes good results, but only where the egoist's own interests are concerned. Moreover, from the perspective of a person trying to make a consequentialist ethical decision, this definition appears to require a kind of omniscience about consequences, which, realistically, one can never attain. After all, how can anyone know ahead of time what all the consequences of every possible action would be, let alone how to balance or compare all these differing consequences?

The most famous attempt to answer questions like these is found in a group of theories called utilitarianism. Historically associated with British philosophers Jeremy Bentham and John Stuart Mill, utilitarianism still attracts considerable support from twentieth-century moral philosophers, though the theory takes many forms. Among the most important are *act utilitarianism* and *rule utilitarianism*. Act utilitarians maintain that an act is morally right (in some versions "obligatory") if it actually (in some versions "predictably") contributes to the greatest happiness (well-being, satisfaction of interests) of the greatest number. Act utilitarianism differs from rule utilitarianism by evaluating each situation individually and on its own. In contrast, rule utilitarians evaluate ethical principles, policies, practices, or rules that have general application, judging them to be ethically justifiable to the extent that they contribute to the greatest happiness of the greatest number. They then apply these principles, practices, or rules in relevant situations, judging actions to be ethical when they follow the rules that generally produce the best consequences, whether or not they do in some particular case. So, for example, an act utilitarian will grant time off on a case-by-case basis, whenever it looks as if the result won't be a problem. But a rule utilitarian will look to the institutional policy and follow it, even if making an exception might work out on a particular occasion.

Rule utilitarians, but not act utilitarians, will go ahead and apply the rules even when they may not produce the best outcome in a particular situation, as long as following the rules generally produces the "greatest happiness." A rule utilitarian might consider it ethically responsible to act on the principle that "honesty is the best policy" even if there are special cases where not telling the exact truth might be more beneficial overall. As we will see, many institutional policies operate this way:

their ethical justification is that these policies may reasonably be assumed to produce the greatest happiness of the greatest number in general, even if on some occasions they generate less than the best outcome. Therefore, the reluctance of decision makers to grant exceptions can have rule-utilitarian roots. Once exceptions are allowed, the force of the rules, practices, or principles that constitute institutional policy is seriously undermined.

> *Managers and policy makers generally think as rule utilitarians. While often unwilling to make exceptions in particular cases, rule utilitarians will modify policies if too many requests occur for exceptions that seem reasonable.*

The phrase "greatest happiness of the greatest number" is easy to misunderstand. As suggested above, the term *happiness* has been construed in a number of different ways. In Benthamite utilitarianism, happiness reduces to pleasure and/or the avoidance of pain, whereas some other versions identify happiness with well-being conceived more broadly or even with the most comprehensive satisfaction of interests at stake in a given situation. By reducing every consequence of any action to its tendency to produce pleasure or pain, Bentham (1789) is thought to have been trying to find a least common denominator that would make possible precise calculations of consequences, even when those consequences are of very differing kinds. In fact, Bentham appears to have thought that he could calculate precisely the ethical values of each possible choice by factoring into his *hedonistic calculus* such considerations as the "purity," "fecundity," and "propinquity" of pleasures and pains, as well as extent, duration, and the number of people (sentient beings, actually) affected by each possibility.[1] But such an approach seems to ignore the possibilities that the proper value of some consequences cannot be reduced to mere pleasure or pain, that they may not share any genuine common denominator, or, as Mill thought, that some consequences are qualitatively better or more worthy than others. Many contemporary utilitarians prefer to weigh competing interests and assign those interests various kinds of differing priorities.

---

[1] Roughly, a "pure" pleasure does not involve any suffering; a hard workout would be impure in this sense. A "fecund" pleasure is one that grows or becomes richer over time, like the appreciation of fine art. A "propinquity" pleasure is immediate, not delayed, like tasting an ice cream cone as opposed to investing money in the stock market. Most general ethics textbooks have extensive discussions of Bentham's hedonistic calculus, though few philosophers now believe it can actually be applied in any but an approximate way.

The question of how to define and then to compare and weigh consequences is, thus, a troubling one for utilitarians. Yet it would be unfair to utilitarianism to make too much of this. Those who reason according to utilitarian patterns normally require not omniscience about consequences but the best rational estimate, recognizing that, even though one may be wrong, one cannot reasonably be considered unethical for not foretelling the future with divine accuracy. And, while precise utilitarian comparisons between consequences for all those whose interests are affected are not likely to achieve scientific accuracy, it is not normally more difficult to make a reasonable assessment of the priority some important issues should have as compared to less important issues. For example, it is intuitively obvious that stopping Smith's arterial hemorrhage outweighs Jones's interest in additional pain relief and that making Jones more comfortable outweighs documenting McCarthy's complaints about the food service.

This example shows something else important about utilitarianism that is often misunderstood. Calculating the balance of consequences is not simply counting up people who are benefited or harmed, so that if there are more who are benefited than there are people whose interests are sacrificed, the action or principle is justified. The extent, duration, amount, and kind of benefits and harms must be considered too. Utilitarians might agree that "the good of the many outweighs the good of the one," but only if the goods in question are similar. No utilitarian would endorse inflicting grave harm on someone merely to provide amusement for a crowd, for example. Utilitarian arguments also can be made to purchase lifesaving equipment when the alternatives offer only convenience or comfort, even if many people enjoy the result. So utilitarians have serious doubts about spending for impressive remodeling or lavish furnishings when there is not enough money to fund basic care or provide needed services, even if only a few people are doing without that care or those services.

Another important aspect of utilitarianism that is sometimes overlooked is that it requires ethical decision makers to consider *all* the consequences for *all* those affected by an action. For Bentham, this "greatest number" means every sentient being, specifically including animals, whose interests (feelings of pleasure or pain) are affected by the proposed course of action. Thus, for Bentham and other utilitarians who share his broad conception of the "greatest number," there are serious ethical questions to be raised about our willingness to sacrifice animals' interests in life and the avoidance of suffering so that we can eat them for dinner or use them in health care training and research (Singer, 1975).

Whether one accepts this broadly inclusive definition of the "greatest number" or not, one of the most important practical problems about utilitarianism is making sure all those whose interests are potentially affected by a course of action are given fair consideration of their interests. One of the best ways to ensure fair consideration is to involve everyone who is affected by a decision in the process of making it. That way, everyone's interests have a spokesperson. When everyone cannot be involved, including representatives of diverse interests in the decision-making process can be helpful. While this approach is not always possible or practical, it is both possible and practical much more often than many decision makers seem to think. For example, as we have already seen, it is quite common for health care institutions (and institutions of other kinds) to weigh their own interests in efficient use of staff time and resources more heavily than they weigh efficient use of patient or client time and resources. What utilitarianism says is that, all other things being equal, everyone's time ought to be given similar weight in calculating ethically appropriate policies. So why not at least involve patient and public representatives in an advisory role when decisions are made that affect them? Such an approach almost always contributes to more responsible decision making and practices.

Here is another common kind of case in which one might be tempted to think in terms of consequences, but without giving suitable consideration to all the consequences for all those affected.

Case 5.2: The Intimidating Lab Technician

Sandy S. is an accurate and fast-working lab technician who does most of the blood work that comes in on her 3:00 to 11:00 shift. She also enjoys her reputation as a tough-as-nails "motorcycle mama." Outside the lab, she's inseparable from her Harley, and the high point of her year is her annual summer trip to Sturgis, South Dakota. Whenever she's not busy, however, Sandy ducks out of the lab; usually she can be found outside the building, smoking cigarettes. And it is not rare for Sandy to have a few beers before coming to work.

Anne K. is a young, straight-laced lab tech who has recently been assigned to Sandy's shift. She is intimidated by Sandy. Without having said so, Sandy and others have made it clear to Anne that she should look the other way concerning Sandy's behavior and even cover for her if the occasion arises. But this afternoon, Sandy seems more than a little inebriated, slurring her words, walking a little stiffly, and speaking in an aggressive tone. Should Anne advise a supervisor about Sandy's condition?

If Anne reasons from consequences in this situation, it will seem obvious on one level that she certainly should advise a supervisor about Sandy's condition. If what Anne suspects about Sandy is true, Sandy poses a considerable risk to the performance of the lab, to her colleagues, and to herself. But other consequences are likely to loom large to Anne. Should she "rat" on Sandy? Sandy might well retaliate against Anne who, after all, is already intimidated by Sandy. Moreover, Sandy is accepted by her colleagues, while Anne is the "new kid on the block." Anne might reasonably expect that her working relationship not only with Sandy, but also with her other colleagues would be jeopardized by informing a supervisor. Moreover, it is unlikely that, if anything did happen as a result of Sandy's inebriation, Anne would be in any way involved or appear accountable.

Under these circumstances it would not be surprising if Anne decided to ignore the problem. But doing so would be hard to justify by consequentialist reasoning or, in fact, by any other reasonable form of ethical thinking. Anne is giving predictable consequences for herself far greater weight than consequences for everyone else. However understandable her feelings may be in this situation, her failure to give adequate weight to the risks for others undermines the ethical justification for her decision.

More specifically, a rule utilitarian would certainly report Sandy, on the grounds that, even if nothing serious happened as a result of this episode, to allow lab staff to work inebriated would not, in general, predictably contribute to the best balance of consequences. And while it is just barely conceivable that an act utilitarian might decide to not report Sandy, the act utilitarian would still have to take extensive steps to make sure that not reporting Sandy this time would really turn out to yield the best balance of consequences, taking into account the likelihood that not reporting Sandy will most likely contribute to future episodes of on-the-job impairment as well as the problems that might occur this time. So it probably would take considerable intellectual acrobatics, if not self-deception, for a utilitarian to justify not reporting Sandy. But it is still worth noticing that act utilitarianism might allow enough "wiggle room" to allow a clearly unprofessional judgment to appear ethical. That is one reason rule-utilitarian reasoning is more commonly characteristic of ethical professional practice.

Utilitarian reasoning often guides institutional decision making, especially where resource allocation is concerned. Consider this letter to Ms. Susan Davis, a public health nurse who has applied to the Newtown Foundation for grant funding of an outreach project.

Case 5.3: The Grant Application

Ms. Susan E. Davis, R.N.
Valley Health Services, Public Health Department
Middleton, Ohio

Dear Ms. Davis:

The Board of Directors of the Newtown Foundation are pleased to inform you that the Foundation has elected to fund your project: "Lead Assessment and Early Childhood Intervention in Inner City Middleton." Detailed information can be found in the accompanying literature. While competition among applicants was keen, the Directors were especially impressed with the number of beneficiaries of your program, the cost-benefit effectiveness to be gained by early intervention versus later crisis management, and the long-lasting benefits to your client population. We wish you every success during the program's implementation phase.

Sincerely,

Ms. Delores Brown, Executive Secretary
The Newtown Foundation

While we do not know what other proposals may have been made to the foundation, this letter strongly suggests that utilitarian considerations determined the outcome of the directors' deliberations. When a cost-benefit analysis yields large numbers of people who will be very positively affected for a long time, utilitarian reasoning would strongly favor that choice. Indeed, so strong is the persuasiveness of utilitarian reasoning, especially where resource-allocation decisions are made, that it is often difficult for decision makers to recognize that other important perspectives should be considered.

It is important to remember that there are other valid ethical perspectives. However persuasive utilitarianism can be, it has some significant limitations; and it is vital to bear these in mind. We have already noted problems in estimating and weighing consequences accurately and in assuring that the comprehensive range of interests of all affected parties is given a fair hearing. Additionally, utilitarianism does not generally guarantee that benefits and sacrifices will be shared equally, nor does it always protect the interests of minorities. Moreover, it does not generally permit special obligations to one's own patients, clients, colleagues, or family, because everyone's similar interests are to be treated similarly.

Unless these factors are considered, utilitarian arguments could lead to hastening the deaths of terminal potential organ donors. Or providing care only for cost-effective, common diseases, while neglecting the problems of people with costly or unpopular afflictions. Or taking unfair advantage of a few people to assure that a larger number could get preferred vacation times. Or abandoning one's own patient whenever it looks as though one might accomplish more with another patient. Or demanding unreasonably self-sacrificing work obligations of employees (because there would almost always be more beneficial things one could be doing rather than, say, buying your children new shoes, to say nothing of attending a concert or working out at the gym: the money could go to famine relief and your time would be better spent caring for the seriously ill).[2]

> *Think like a utilitarian for a moment. How might a utilitarian argue for hastening the deaths of organ donors? Or for including benefits for common diseases but excluding benefits for rare ones? Or for loading up the least senior staff people during the summer so that the majority of more senior staff can have preferred vacation time? Or for mandatory overtime? Is there any merit to these arguments?*

In summary, despite its problems and critics, utilitarianism is certainly one of the most commonly practiced forms of ethical reasoning. This is especially true in public policy areas, partly because the approach seems so similar to democratic procedures like voting: each person's similar interests count similarly, and the goal is to produce the best outcome for the largest number. Utilitarian thinking is also commonly used in resource-allocation debates because it is so similar to the kind of straightforward cost-benefit analysis commonly used in managerial decision making. Properly conducted, utilitarian reasoning can be an important contribution to the resolution of ethical dilemmas. But it is also subject to misapplications and distortions; and, like all reasoning, it has limitations. To avoid these, it is important to make sure that all the affected parties and their interests are given fair consideration, that important principles and responsibilities do not get lost, and that the interests of minorities are adequately safeguarded. One useful way to overcome its limitations is to involve all those who are affected in the decision; but, when this is impossible, thorough consideration is crucial.

---

[2] Whether utilitarianism creates insupportable obligations is an issue contemporary utilitarians take very seriously indeed. Peter Singer's vision of what utilitarianism requires in *Practical Ethics* (Cambridge: Cambridge University Press, 1979) certainly strikes many (but not all) readers as insupportable. Among the most influential critics of utilitarianism along these lines is Shelly Kagan, in *The Limits of Morality* (Oxford: Clarendon Press, 1989).

QUESTIONS FOR DISCUSSION

1. *Case 5.4: Justifying Budget Requests*—As director of the occupational therapy department, you have been invited to join other directors to work out this year's budget. Your top priority is an elevator-equipped van, to be used to acclimate clients to a large range of tasks of ordinary living. It appears that the main alternative to funding the van is to spend a similar amount of money on a cryosurgical device to be used in a few rare cases of liver surgery. Give a utilitarian argument in favor of spending the money on the van as opposed to the cryosurgical machine. Can a utilitarian argument be given in favor of the cryosurgical device? Explain.

2. *Case 5.5: Is Our Treatment of Animals Speciesist?*—Australian philosopher Peter Singer (1975, 1979) has argued that to ignore or devalue animal suffering to achieve human interests can be a kind of ethical blindness similar to racism. That is, just as a racist irrationally sacrifices the interests of those of other races to benefit himself or his own race, so, Singer argues, human beings act as immoral "speciesists" when they sacrifice the interests of animals to achieve human interests that are not at least equally important. How do you think a consistent utilitarian would argue that each of the following can be immoral or unethical? Do you agree? Why or why not?

    a. Placing concentrated solutions of painful, blinding chemicals in the eyes of rabbits in order to develop new cosmetics.

    b. Raising, buying, and eating veal. Other animals?

    c. Crushing the skulls of monkeys in order to study the effects of concussions.

    d. Deliberately infecting chimpanzees with HIV in order to test possible AIDS treatments.

3. Recall case 1.5, in which Alice P., who has used up all her personal leave time, is tempted to call in ill in order to take her daughter to audition for the role of Clara in the ballet *The Nutcracker.* Suppose you are Alice's supervisor, and Alice is now on the telephone; she is asking that you grant her one more day of personal leave, even though Alice knows she has exhausted her allotment. You think you and your staff probably could stretch to cover for Alice, given today's fairly light work load. How would a rule utilitarian probably respond to Alice's request? How might an act utilitarian justify granting Alice's request? What do you think is the most ethically responsible thing to do? Why?

REASONING FROM PRINCIPLES
(DEONTOLOGICAL ETHICS)

Case 5.6: Cost-Effectiveness Isn't Everything

Jack M., CEO of Community Hospital, is faced with continuing financial difficulties due, in large measure, to the hospital's elderly and impoverished client population. On examining the figures developed by the finance department, Jack discovers that the least-cost-effective services provided by the hospital are long-term chronic care (LTC) for elderly patients and obstetrics (OB). LTC is unprofitable because most patients are covered by Medicare, and the reimbursement level is below the hospital's costs. OB is unprofitable because it requires a number of staff who are then unavailable for anything else, because the aging community uses the service less and less, and because those who are using it are either underinsured or covered only by Medicaid, which, like Medicare, reimburses only about 80 percent of costs. The appeal of dropping these programs is considerable, but Jack is acutely uncomfortable about depriving the community of these services. No matter how cost-effective it would be, Jack concludes, it would be wrong to drop these programs because, he says, "Community Hospital has a responsibility to this area that transcends our bottom line. We're just going to have to find other avenues to strengthen our financial base."

In this situation, Jack is not reasoning as a utilitarian or, in fact, any kind of consequentialist. Instead, he is taking certain responsibilities as morally obligatory regardless of their consequences. Any similar approach to ethical decision making, in which decisions are based on duties, obligations, principles, or responsibilities that are taken to be basic irrespective of consequences, is a type of *deontological ethics*, or reasoning from principle. In health care, actions based on the mission of the facility would be considered principle-based.

There are almost certainly far too many deontological principles to list completely, even though many people think of ethics in just this way, as a catalog of rules to apply to every situation. Here are some examples of deontological principles: do not abandon a patient; first, do no harm; always respect patient confidentiality. The Ten Commandments, "love thy neighbor as thyself," and other ethical directives based on religion are deontological principles; in fact, "divine command theories" are among the earliest ethical approaches. Respect the humanity (autonomy) of other persons; treat people fairly; treat people justly—each of these is a commonly accepted, even basic, ethical principle. Act as you might consistently wish all other similarly situated persons to act as well; treat people only as ends in themselves, never as means—both of these principles are associated with the influential German philosopher Immanuel Kant. And many more principles might also be listed.

Although principle-based reasoning assumes that an action is good in and of itself, the approach still requires identification and validation of and agreement on what the appropriate principles, duties, and responsibilities are. Partly because there seem to be so many candidates for the list of ethical principles, philosophers have tried to determine which are the most fundamental or basic and then to derive other principles from that fundamental or basic list. In fact, it is probably fair to say that the most difficult problem for deontological approaches to ethical decision making is identifying, validating, and securing agreement about the importance and priority of the various principles, duties, and responsibilities that might be taken to be basic. Many historical sources or theories of validation for deontological principles have been given; however, none has achieved anything like complete or universal acceptance.

Many competing arguments have been made that we know what the deontological principles are and why they are valid. First, people argue, these principles are consistent with God's will. But how do we know what God's will is? Recall our earlier discussion of problems resolving professional ethical issues by means of religious ethics: there we argued that, given the extreme diversity of differing religious traditions and our pluralistic—even secular—society, we are wise to avoid specifically religious justifications for professional ethical decisions.

Second, some have argued that these principles are derived from human nature. That is, principles like "respect people's autonomy" derive from the very nature of human beings, which is to exercise free self-determination. Others, including St. Thomas Aquinas, believed that ethical norms could be derived from "natural law," the patterns of behavior that lead to fulfillment of the purpose or goal for which nature or God intends us. But empiricists and other critics often deny that human beings have a determinate nature or, indeed, that there is anything like a natural law from which ethical norms can be derived. Even if we could somehow know what the very nature of human beings is, it is not self-evident that we have an ethical responsibility to assure that what is natural has free scope for expression. Besides, what if human nature is not to exercise free self-determination, but rather to dominate or even to overpower and take advantage of others? What if it is natural to procreate as often and with as many partners as possible? If human nature is not benign, we might actually have an ethical obligation to resist it.

Third, some argue that deontological principles are consistent with human rights. But, as we have already seen, it is frequently difficult to determine who has what rights, or which rights take priority over which. Moreover, it may be that rights theories depend on assumptions concerning human nature—that the rights one has depend on what is required to be "fully human" or to meet what are taken to be "basic human needs." But, again, what human nature is or what basic human needs are seems deeply bound up with culturally or socially relative assumptions, rather than any genuinely independent scientific evidence.

Fourth, some argue that basic ethical principles may be known intuitively (or through people's consciences). Supporters of this view often point out the widespread uniformity of ethical principles and practices and call the sense of right and wrong associated with this awareness "conscience." But what people's consciences tell them is apparently very much conditioned by one's society. And certainly people have felt conscientiously justified in doing obviously unethical and immoral things. Accordingly, "intuitionism" is vulnerable to our earlier discussion of problems resolving professional ethical issues by means of social relativism or following one's emotions.

Among the most important deontological philosophers is Immanuel Kant (Frankena, 1973). Roughly, Kant and his followers propose that, instead of deriving ethical principles from a determinate human nature, morality should be derived from the dictates of reason: from considerations of noncontradiction and generalization, for example. While we cannot explore his highly technical ideas of "contradiction" and "generalization" here, the basic ideas might be put this way. Right actions are those that are motivated by considerations of duty. Duties, in turn, are consistent with principles that are equally applicable to anyone in a similar situation; wrong actions are those that seem to create a tension between what we would like to do and what we would like others to do in similar circumstances. Thus there is something contradictory about my expecting others to tell the truth but considering it all right for me to lie, or about my expecting others to respect my private property but considering it all right for me to steal theirs or to trespass. And, Kant thinks, once we recognize that ethical principles apply equally to everyone, we must recognize that each person has similar moral standing, that each person deserves equal respect as a person, a being capable of self-determination (autonomy), and therefore as someone who must not be treated merely as a means to accomplish other purposes, even if the result is a generally beneficial outcome (Frankena, 1973).

Although they are not easy for most people to understand or appreciate fully, Kant's ideas have been influential, even on people who do not share his ethical theory. Respect for the humanity or human dignity of people is widespread, as is the idea that ethical principles apply impersonally to everyone, even among people who reason in ways unrelated to Kantian thinking. Rule utilitarianism, for example, can be seen as combining the consequentialist concern about beneficial outcomes with an emphasis on generalization and protection for persons that parallel Kant's. So one does not have to understand and accept all of Kant's ideas to recognize important themes.

At the same time, Kant's version of deontological ethics has many critics. Much of the persuasiveness of Kant's theory depends on doubtful assumptions about human rationality, as if reasoning were one straightforward process shared by all of humanity and entirely divorced from the concrete immediacy of life and its decisions. Why should we think that everyone reasons alike or that duties are always universal rather than specific to individuals and circumstances?[3] Also, people are motivated by many kinds of considerations, and often those considerations are mixed in ways impossible to separate; why suppose that anything less than a pure motivation of duty deprives an action of its ethical character? Moreover, whether something seems contradictory may depend on how one describes the situation. I might very well decide that anyone in my special and peculiar circumstances ought to lie, steal, or trespass, but no one else should; and that might not seem contradictory at all, at least to me.

Some philosophers have tried to locate the heart of deontological principle in respect for the humanity, or human dignity, of those affected. Sometimes "personhood" rather than "humanity" is used to capture this idea because the heart of what is worthy of respect is thought to be that complex cluster of features that makes us "persons" rather than simply biologically human. Such features as the capacity for rationality, self-concept, interpersonal relationships, self-determination, and the potential for transformation have been popular choices for the locus of what is distinctively valuable about persons.[4]

But there is little agreement on what it is about persons that entitles them to respect or what respect for human dignity actually requires.

---

[3] The idea that rationality is not one universal and timeless procedure of thought, or that an ethical principle like justice is not always conceived in precisely the same way, does not have to lead to any of the ethically suspect forms of relativism we criticized in Chapter 4. There are many other alternatives between blindness to the diversity of human thought and indefensible relativism. For a fascinating analysis of this issue, see Alasdair MacIntyre, *Whose Justice? Which Rationality?* (Notre Dame, Ind.: Notre Dame University Press, 1988).

[4] Jane English's article "Abortion and the Concept of a Person" is a wonderful formulation of this idea, partly because it does not oversimplify. Originally published in the *Canadian Journal of Philosophy,* vol. 5, no. 2 (October 1975), the article has been widely republished.

Moreover, many people consider that we ought to extend respect for human dignity to people who lack the capacity for rationality, self-concept, interpersonal relationships, or self-determination, such as anencephalic infants, stroke victims, and perhaps even the dead. Furthermore, many animals, including those humans seem willing to abuse as they would not abuse other humans, appear to exhibit far more "person characteristics" than many humans do. For example, we run medical tests on animals far more "personlike" than many humans. Have we any moral right to do so? Or should we extend this kind of respect for "persons" to nonhuman persons?

All this may seem unnecessarily complicated. As mentioned earlier, the health care professions are themselves historically committed to a number of principles, most famously "First, do no harm," but also principles of nonabandonment, beneficence, and confidentiality, among others. A number of prominent hospital organizations even state their commitments to certain guiding principles in their mission statements, on their logos, and elsewhere. For example, Mercy Health Services officially rests on the principles of "service, justice, human dignity, mercy, and [options] for the poor" (McAuley, circa 1831). Why not simply appeal to such principles as these, which enjoy such widespread support within health care circles?

As a practical matter, arguing for an ethical decision based on principles to which an institution is officially committed is a powerful strategy. Sometimes it may be the most effective approach when trying to win over people who are otherwise sensitive only to cost-benefit analyses or effects on their own departments. But from a larger, ethical theoretical point of view, using such principles as these does not explain how they are to be prioritized when they conflict or even how they are to be applied in particular situations. Moreover, an institution's commitment to such principles, however admirable, does not commit everyone else to those principles, certainly not patients and families and often not even employees. Even more important from a theoretical point of view, it is not clear what justifies these principles, what these principles ultimately rest on—whether God's will, respect for human dignity, or something else. So traditional health care principles and even official institutional commitments can be practically useful and still leave many important questions unanswered.

Yet reasoning from such principles as these has many advantages. Among these are that principled reasoning avoids many of the problems of consequentialist theories by protecting individuals against the tyranny of the group, respecting an irreducible minimum of human value regardless of possible gains, promoting justice, yielding minimally fair (or just) distributions of benefits, limiting sacrifices, and promoting respect for persons.

Besides, on consideration, it seems obvious and correct to most people that certain actions are morally wrong no matter how good their consequences might be. For example, most people would agree that even if a slave-holding society were better off on the whole than it would be without slaves, even with the misery of the slaves figured in, that fact would still not be enough to make slavery morally acceptable. Framing and executing an innocent person in order to deter others from committing crimes would clearly be unjust, even if it benefited society greatly. Hastening the deaths of terminal patients in order to harvest their organs for transplantation would clearly violate even the most minimal principles of ethical practice, no matter how much good might be done for the transplant recipients. Even the most outspoken utilitarians, like Bentham and Mill, seem to some critics to covertly depend on certain nonutilitarian norms or principles to make their consequential calculations be consistent with principled moral judgments.

Because of all the problems with defending and justifying principles and because of the pervasiveness of consequentialist reasoning, especially where financial issues and public policy are concerned, it is easy to be swept along and not give sufficient consideration to such issues as fairness, justice, respect for autonomy, and deontological principles generally. We cannot emphasize strongly enough that health care professionals have a crucial role as patient/client advocates, defending their interests against what might be expedient or cost-effective. The best weapon we have to oppose a heartless commitment to the bottom line regardless of what happens to individual people is to argue that, even if some course of action is cost-effective, it is still wrong if it is also unjust or unfair.

Once more, these arguments are strengthened when institutions have made explicit commitments to values such as human dignity, mercy, justice, quality care, or options for the indigent. Many health care institutions do have policy statements committing them to respect for such values as these; it is very useful to find out what they are.[5] Such values are deontological principles that can be opposed to consequentialist reasoning to protect individual patients and clients.

---

[5] In fact, current guidelines from the Joint Commission on Accreditation of Healthcare Organizations for 1996 require a number of explicit commitments to principles, rules, rights, and responsibilities.

A FEW WORDS ABOUT THE RIGHT TO LIFE

One very outspoken advocacy group that employs a commitment to ethical principles in a politically influential way is a collection of organizations often called the "Right to Life movement." The principle at the heart of the ethical stance most often associated with right to life is that innocent human life is sacred from the moment of conception. Applying this principle has led to consistent opposition to all forms of abortion and to opposition to other procedures, such as in vitro fertilization and preimplantation selection, which involve the intentional destruction of human embryos.

We will not address questions about the ethics of abortion here. However, right to life offers a case study of how principled reasoning can be powerfully influential, yet leave people vulnerable to certain kinds of criticisms. The seemingly simple principle that all innocent human life is sacred from the moment of conception appeals to many because it avoids the vague and arbitrary effort to draw lines between acceptable and unacceptable forms of killing. However, there is no identifiable moment at which conception occurs. It is a process that takes at least twenty-four hours (if conception is identified with syngamy), but that may not be completed until fourteen days later, when the possibility of splitting into identical twins has been lost. There are also questions associated with the idea of "innocence" and questions about the religious commitment that might be implicit in calling human life "sacred" (because one can certainly take a right-to-life position without making any particular religious commitment).

Over and above these problems, advocates of the right to life find themselves with a fundamental difficulty in arguing their case that can be characteristic of deontological reasoning more generally. The problem is that right-to-life advocates regard the sanctity of innocent human life as a (perhaps, the) fundamental ethical principle. So, when asked by others "Why do you think that ending an innocent human life is always morally indefensible?" the only answers are to repeat the principle that innocent human life is sacred or to insist that the answer is obvious or that the principle is a self-justifying ethical fact. But repeating the principle does not explain why it is true. Insisting the principle is obvious ignores the fact that it is not obvious to those asking for a justification. And claiming that the principle is self-justifying, an ethical fact, looks, to others who do not agree, like a tacit admission that the principle has no justification or at least no justification that is intelligible to the unconverted.

From the right-to-life perspective, of course, people who are seriously unable to see why innocent human life is sacred are exactly on a par with people who are unable to see what's so bad about the Jewish

Holocaust during World War II or who look on entertained while a molester rapes a schoolchild. That is, from the right-to-life perspective, those who are unable to see the truth of the "innocent life is sacred" principle either suffer from a serious form of moral blindness or, worse, become demonized, as if perversion rather than blindness were the real problem. Such accusations, or even such suspicions, do nothing to promote mutual understanding.

But they reveal a problem at the heart of deontological reasoning: unless there is broad agreement on fundamental ethical principles to begin with—or unless agreement on specific principles can be derived from fundamental agreement on such deeper and more general ethical foundations as respect for human dignity, the importance of fairness, or something else with similar ethical power—reasoning from principle can degenerate into hurling labels at each other or demonizing each other. Such a situation is certainly not helpful even when it is not covertly destructive. So it is important to try to secure agreement about the principles on which principled reasoning will ultimately be based.

QUESTIONS FOR DISCUSSION

1. *Case 5.7: Home-Care Patient's Insurance Has Run Out*—Valley Home Care has been providing twice-weekly visits by an R.N. and daily visits by a nursing assistant to Francine R., who is largely incapacitated by multiple sclerosis. Confined to her bed, Francine is neglected by her husband, who often allowed her to go unfed or to lie in her own feces for days at a time. Visiting nurses also suspect he abuses Francine sexually, though she will not confirm this, and her catheter is often pulled out when they arrive. The couple's insurance will no longer reimburse care for the catheter, nor for the other home-care visits. The visiting nurses and aides are extremely reluctant to cease their visits, knowing that Francine is likely to be at serious risk. But the finance department is also reluctant to authorize continued care without prospect for reimbursement. "What kind of precedent are you setting here?" they ask. How could deontological principles be raised to argue in favor of continuing care for Francine? Are there other ways in which finance's concerns might be met?

2. About 44 million Americans, a large portion of them employed, lack health insurance and therefore lack access to many services. With which deontological principles does this situation conflict? Is there any plausible ethical argument to allow this situation to go on?

3. *Case 5.8: Vacation Scheduling Priorities*—You are a negotiator for the upcoming Service International Employees Union contract with River City Medical Center. Among the contentious issues raised by union members is the matter of vacation schedules. For example, while each employee is limited to two weeks during May through September, and no more than three R.N.s and two L.P.N.s on a given unit can take the same week off, requests are currently filled according to seniority, with the most senior R.N. getting first choice until all R.N. requests have been filled, then the most senior L.P.N., and so on. Low-seniority nurses object because they often do not receive vacations at preferred times, and sometimes receive no vacations at all. L.P.N.s object because they feel discriminated against. But senior R.N.s argue that since they've not only "put in their time," but also have higher levels of responsibility, they have earned "first dibs."

   How does this situation illustrate a conflict between what might be considered fair versus what might be considered just? Is there a utilitarian justification for a procedure like this? What do you think the most ethically responsible vacation assignment procedure would be? Why?

CHAPTER SIX

Professionalism, Virtue Ethics, and Feminism

Although consequentialist and principled (deontological) perspectives are the leading ethical theories among many philosophers, other approaches are attracting considerable interest. Underlying this development is the sense that neither a strict consequentialist nor a strict deontological theory really captures a sufficiently rich and plausible conception of ethics, either as a model of professional ethics or as a way of living. Moreover, these patterns of reasoning have seemed to many critics to be much more characteristic of masculine problem solving than of feminine approaches to value conflicts. As a result, many philosophers have suggested that emphasis on consequentialist and principled reasoning needs to be balanced with other defensible patterns of ethical thinking.

These feelings are shared by many health care professionals, who are called on to be more than shrewd calculators of the greatest happiness of the greatest number or principled practitioners respecting the autonomy of their patients while seeking to be just and fair. To many, approaches like these seem sterile and insensitive to the human needs and interests involved in value conflicts. Something more is needed. Health care professionals might call what is needed "true professionalism," traditional ethics combined with a sensitivity to human feelings. Among philosophers, these kinds of theories, focused on traits of character and personality and informed by feminist sensibilities, combine what is called virtue ethics with feminist ethical theory. However, philosophers do not necessarily link virtue ethics with feminist ethics. Historically, they developed quite separately, with virtue ethics originating among classical Greek philosophers, and feminist ethics becoming an explicit movement only recently. We begin with the ideas of professionalism and virtue and then turn to feminist ethics.

> Virtue ethics *is a pattern of ethical reasoning emphasizing responsible, admirable traits of character rather than judgments about particular actions.*
>
> Feminist ethics *is a pattern of ethical reasoning emphasizing the importance of traditionally feminine values such as relationship and caring in ethical decision making.*

PROFESSIONALISM AND VIRTUE

What is it to be truly professional? What is it to be truly virtuous? It is not simply to think or act in responsible ways, although true professionals normally do think and act responsibly. Nor is it merely to be fully acculturated to the institutional environment in which one practices. Rather, it is to be a certain kind of person—respectful and appreciative of the traditions of one's discipline, yet also compassionate, wise, competent, caring: the kind of person others can count on.[1] It is to be a person who exhibits an inner confidence and stability, as if at peace with oneself. It is to be the kind of person who intuitively understands and acts in ways appropriately "responsive to all the morally relevant considerations in their right proportions," whether or not all those considerations would be easy, or even possible, to articulate to other members of an ethics committee (Ross, 1939).

Aristotle in ancient Greece and Confucius in China, as well as many other moral philosophers ancient and modern, have recognized that becoming such a person as we have described here is a project for our entire lives, even though some people are already very far along. But

---

[1] As we shall see, exactly what should be considered a virtue, or, more specifically, what are the moral and what are the nonmoral virtues, is not an obvious matter. Richard Brandt, for example, says that "some action-explaining traits like ambition, industry, and curiosity, which have all the features mentioned earlier as essential for traits of character (stability and relative permanence in normal frames of mind, being intrinsic desires), would hardly be called virtues, at least moral ones." And, later on, he adds "enterprise, orderliness, self-reliance, and independence" to his list of beneficial traits which, however, he would not call morally good (Richard B. Brandt, "W. K. Frankena and Ethics of Virtue," in *The Monist*, La Salle, IL 61301, 1981). We accept the ideas that stability, relative permanence, and being a desire or aversion not simply derivable from or reducible to deontological principles or consequences may all be aspects of virtues. But we think the distinction between moral and nonmoral virtues is not of much practical importance in this context. And we will shortly explore criteria for identifying what should be counted as virtues.

perhaps it would be useful to try to illustrate the differences between how someone reasoning according to the professional virtues might address an ethical dilemma and how a consequentialist or principled analyst might approach the matter.

Case 6.1: Medication Errors Threaten Job Loss

Sandy R., R.N., has been a capable nurse whose generous nature and outgoing personality have made her popular with her patients and colleagues. About two months ago, however, her husband filed for divorce and custody of their two children because, he told Sandy, "we just can't compete with your job; you just don't have anything left for us when you get home; we're just your codependency, not a family." Although her colleagues try to be supportive, Sandy has become extremely depressed; and, probably because of this, she has made several medication errors.

Ann J. is doing quality assurance reviews and has discovered that Sandy incorrectly transcribed a physician's order for morphine as 15mg q4h instead of 5mg q4h. Two doses were given at the higher level, but Ann checked on the patient and assessed him as having had no ill effects from the error. Seeing Sandy in the hall, Ann went with her to the conference room and explained the problem.

When confronted, Sandy fell apart. In tears, she begged Ann to conceal the error because if it became known, hospital policy would require that she be suspended or even fired for having made more than three medication errors within a six-month period. But her upcoming divorce hearing makes it crucial that she have continuing, stable employment; otherwise she will probably lose custody of her children. What should Ann do?

The issue confronting Ann can be analyzed in different ways. As an act utilitarian, for example, Ann might try to determine which course of action open to her is likely to produce the greatest happiness for those affected; she might decide to conceal the error while, however, carefully avoiding assignments for Sandy that place patients at risk, at least until after the divorce hearing. As a reasoner from principle, the issue is more difficult to sort because it is not clear what all the relevant principles are. But it would not be surprising if Ann decided that protecting patients is the higher-priority value at stake in this situation and reported Sandy, perhaps with a recommendation that the suspension be mitigated under the circumstances.

But to analyze this situation along either of these lines (or, in fact, to analyze it at all) might also be seen as morally insensitive, or callous.

What about Sandy's obvious suffering? What about the terrible dilemma she finds herself in, struggling to salvage at least something of her family and, at the same time, to maintain her career? Of course Ann must safeguard Sandy's patients. But a person who fails to empathize deeply enough with Sandy's conflicted predicament demonstrates a moral failing too—a failure in virtue, a failure to be the right kind of person. Intuitively, Ann might feel this situation as a conflict between competence and integrity on the one hand and her feelings of compassion and concern for a friend on the other. That is, Ann may feel pulled toward reporting Sandy by her respect for capable practice and by her own sense of honesty, but also pulled toward trying to protect Sandy by her friendship for a colleague and her ability to empathize with Sandy's fears.

Classical virtue ethics emphasizes the importance of developing moral character in people so that when they are confronted with specific moral dilemmas, their responses will flow naturally from settled moral dispositions or habits. So, for example, when a specific situation calls for courage, a virtuous person will already have trained his or her character so that the strength of character that is needed to act courageously is already there to be called on. But how do we develop courage? The short answer is, people develop virtues by acting as if they are already virtuous. People develop courage and the other moral virtues by setting themselves challenges that are increasingly difficult and then acting virtuously in those situations. And as people are ready for more and more difficult challenges and meet them, they increasingly become the kind of person who can deal with the moral problems life throws at them; they become virtuous.

Virtue ethics theorists are not suggesting that decent people can never fail or that a (normally) virtuous person will never act badly. Virtue ethicists emphasize only that when people do fail to meet a challenge to their moral character, they have to face that fact, make what amends they can, and try again another time. One action "out of character" doesn't amount to a lifetime failure to be ethically responsible. Living an ethically responsible life is a lifelong process of moral development with the long-term goal of yielding a good life while recognizing the frailties of human nature and the misfortunes that can derail even the best of intentions and efforts. However, to persist in failing to act well under trying circumstances or to continue in patterns of behavior that are insensitive, cowardly, or dishonest, will make a person insensitive, cowardly, or dishonest. People are as responsible for those morally ugly traits of character (the vices) that they develop in themselves as they are for those morally admirable ones (the virtues) they manage to achieve.

An ethics of the virtues yields a much-enriched conception of ethics and morality, helping to counteract the diminishment of these ideas that is widespread in contemporary culture. Whereas principled and consequentialist reasoning methods judge moral actions by means of public criteria that may seem simplistic, classical virtue theory emphasizes the importance of an interior dimension of moral decision making and an appreciation for the immense complexity of issues as real life presents them. Whereas much contemporary moral theory treats moral choices as isolated events in people's lives, classical virtue theory treats the entirety of our lives, personalities, and ways of living as an indissoluble whole. Virtues are not left at the workplace; they are part and parcel of our personalities, with us always. So virtue ethics is not just something we do at work. It's the whole of life.

Now, what exactly is a virtue? Providing a clear and universally accepted definition may not be possible. We tend to recognize virtues in the actions or personalities of people whom we admire and have confidence in. Examples of virtues that are widely recognized include wisdom, courage, compassion, generosity, gratitude, honor, and self-respect. Examples of vices include hypocrisy, self-deception, jealousy, laziness, gluttony, and narcissism. But there is more to virtue than merely commanding admiration and confidence.

First, virtues are settled or habitual traits of character. No one would be described as a courageous person who, though a mouse most of the time, once in a great while managed to stand up to an intimidating coworker. Second, virtues work together to contribute to living a truly human life well. Wise, courageous, compassionate people are also typically happy with their lives. In contrast, excessive self-sacrifice or obsessive cleanliness, which are not normally considered virtues, often lead people to be much less happy.

Virtues are expressed but not completely defined through individual actions. So someone could act generously whenever generosity is called for, yet not really be generous if, for example, his or her motives were entirely self-serving, underlain with bitter resentment each time. Virtues have to be developed, cultivated, and maintained through vigilant self-appraisal and hard work. So, for example, being tall would not be a virtue, even if it was beneficial, since it requires no effort on the part of anyone who is tall. But being truthful would normally be a virtue, in part because we often have strong desires not to tell the whole truth or even part of it. The fact that training oneself to be virtuous does require effort is connected to another fact about virtues, that cultivating and possessing them amounts to a kind of self-mastery. Here, again, is the point made earlier, that true professionals seem at peace with themselves, but not through smugness or self satisfaction; the sense of being at peace comes from truly being a good person.

Many, but perhaps not all, virtues are, at least to some extent, independent of specific times and social arrangements. For example, it is difficult to find a culture or society—or even a person—that has admired cowardice or unkindness, perhaps because many, if not all, of the virtues may be necessary or extremely helpful in any durable form of social life.[2] But it would give a false impression to suggest too strongly that the concept of virtue is entirely unanimous. Instead, it is probably closer to the truth to suggest that at least some virtues are connected with one's position or responsibilities. Thus, for example, it may be virtuous for an accrediting investigator to be inquisitive, blunt, or reluctant to take explanations at face value, but it would not be virtuous in a colleague or friend who had no reason for suspicion.

This line of thought raises interesting possibilities. First, if the most important virtues (or the virtues per se) depend at least to some extent on one's position or responsibilities, then professionalism may link up with one's role in a more ethically acceptable way than the minimal role-based ethics rejected in Chapter 2. In fact, some have suggested that the specific content of a professional ethics of virtues may well be derivable at least in part from a rich notion of the functions of the relevant profession. That is, while many virtues belong in a list of professional virtues irrespective of the profession in question merely because they are human virtues, some virtues will be more important than others because of specific obligations and roles in a specific profession. But we would not want to go too far in this direction. In this era of increasingly interdepartmental case management, when members of the health professions must come to regard each other as colleagues (and also live up to the demands of collegiality), older stereotypes of, for example, abject subordination to doctors are no longer viable, regardless of role expectations.

Second, virtues cannot always be articulated as principles or consequences, because they are often closer to feelings or ways of being than to reasoning. The influence of compassion, say, or respect for competence may be sensed in ways that defy full explanation to others. While an ethic of pure feeling was rejected earlier because of the variability and

---

[2] But not all cultures have admired all the same traits. Much disagreement can be set aside because of differing ideas of who has moral standing. Thus, while mercy toward one's fellow citizens is a virtue, mercy toward someone thought to merit mercilessness—an unrepentant convicted murderer, say—might not be considered a virtue. But at least some philosophers point to the possibility of much deeper differences. See, for example, Alasdair MacIntyre's *A Short History of Ethics* (1966), *After Virtue* (1989), and *Whose Justice? Which Rationality?* (1981).

ethical indefensibility of (some) feelings, one of the most important goals of studying ethics is to sensitize people (people's feelings) to ethical issues they might not otherwise notice or be able to address. A sensitive, compassionate health professional may not be able to explain exactly what is bothersome about a situation in which there are important ethical tensions, but will nevertheless be able to feel and draw attention to the problem.

In Ann's case, she might experience a strong sense of solidarity with Sandy and against administrators who would single-mindedly apply rules suspending Sandy without compassionate regard for her circumstances. However, to allow one's feelings for a close colleague to turn the situation into an "us versus them" confrontation would not be useful or responsible and would certainly not exemplify the broadest interpretation of professionalism. Alternatively, Ann's sense that there is something ethically troubling about the application of rules without regard for their individual circumstances and costs is consistent with the ethical sensitivity that is an important aspect of professionalism. Perhaps the best solution here is to negotiate a reduced or supervised workload for Sandy while her problems are resolved. Such an approach would blend the virtues of compassion, camaraderie, competence, and concern for quality care.

In the end, such a balance of virtues, together with the wisdom necessary to express them, is the goal of an ethic of professional virtues. When it is achieved—and remember that this is a lifelong project—such an ethic can yield a sense of confidence about our own lives without smugness or self-righteousness—a sense of having done our best and being at peace with that. The underlying intuition of an ethics of virtue is that, although applying ethics to modern life includes learning to form and defend responsible positions on moral dilemmas, it is not enough to be shrewd in calculating consequences or quick to identify the most important principles at stake. What is needed is not merely to *act* ethically, but to *be a good person* in both our personal and professional lives. Placing our professional activities in the context of our whole lives rather than isolating our professional life from our private life can lead to a more satisfyingly integrated way of living. The sense of satisfaction that derives from true professionalism offers a way to understand and organize our experiences, to act, and to give our lives meaning. Moreover, an ethics of virtues provides a worthwhile alternative to the essentially meaningless "self-help book" prescription for "being the best you can be" by providing specific norms for human excellence.

An ethics of professionalism is not without problems, of course. As in Ann's case, being virtuous does not necessarily tell someone what to do in a particular situation. And, more generally, "fleshing out" any particular virtue remains difficult unless we fall back on definitions in terms of actions or function. But defining virtues in terms of actions threatens to reduce an ethics of virtue back to the mere appraisal of actions rather than of character. And defining virtues in terms of function presupposes that role-based ethics is sufficient to define desirable traits of character, a position we have already criticized. Neither explains why virtues are morally good.

Besides, not everyone would agree that the effect of an ethics of virtue, of seeing our whole lives as an indissoluble unity, is a good thing. As observed earlier, there is considerable resistance to the idea that anyone's way of living is open to ethical scrutiny. Much of this resistance is due to contemporary society's stress on tolerance, cultural and moral pluralism, respect for privacy, and a large sphere of personal preferences. Besides, any reasonably complete ethics of virtue is quite difficult to practice, and most yield fairly negative self-evaluations at least some of the time. Most of us, after all, are not always as courageous, compassionate, or wise as we ought to be. In a society in which "feeling good about ourselves" has virtually unquestioned importance, modes of thinking that do not yield this result are widely resisted. Further, there is a widespread feeling that one's private life ought somehow to be off-limits for ethical criticism, provided that one's professional behavior is exemplary.

Virtue ethics rejects this segregation of life into personal and professional realms in an especially forthright way. No one can be a compassionate person who "turns it on" at the beginning of a shift and "turns it off" again at the end. Such a person is merely acting compassionate, rather than being compassionate. This is the behavior of a phony, and patients and clients pick up on and dislike such behavior. From the perspective of virtue ethics, virtues need to be genuine, not simulated; they need to be part of who we are as people rather than appearances we put on for certain occasions.

QUESTIONS FOR DISCUSSION

1. *Case 6.2: Staffing Shortages*—Jenny is the nursing supervisor on duty at Metropolitan Hospital, responsible for staffing all the units for the next shift. She knows that the critical care unit requires two licensed personnel at all times, as well as no more than a 1:2 nurse-patient ratio. Three nurses are scheduled, and census is low—only three patients, of whom two are stable. Meanwhile, there is a staffing crisis on two other floors, where one unit is two nurses

short and the other is one nurse short. Jenny could easily pull two nurses from the critical care area, send them to the units that are scrambling, and replace one with a nursing assistant (unlicensed) without running any real patient-care risks. Are there any ethical issues involved in this situation? How should such situations be handled?

2. *Case 6.3: The Christmas Party*—The surgical services department was excited about the upcoming Christmas party. This year's planning committee had approached all the surgeons and they had donated generously. A hall had been booked, and decorations were going to be very special this year: it would be fun, but the real meaning of Christmas would not be lost. The menu would be lavish, featuring honey-baked ham, barbequed spareribs, and stuffed pork chops. Amy, one member of the planning committee, was glad she was the scheduler for surgical services, since she didn't know of any other department that had such wonderful holiday parties. Are there any ethical issues involved in this situation? How should such situations be handled? (Remember, several of the staff are almost certainly Jewish, Hindu, or Muslim.)

3. *Case 6.4: The Unresponsive Surgeon*—Dr. Islam was the trauma surgeon on call when a 25-year-old male arrived with injury to the abdomen. The patient was in shock and had received four units of blood, yet the bleeding had not been controlled. Dr. Islam asked that Dr. Steinberg, the house "expert" in trauma management, be paged and asked to assist him. The nurse in the operating room paged Dr. Steinberg repeatedly, but Steinberg did not respond. After five hours of surgery, Dr. Islam packed the abdominal cavity with sponges, made a temporary closure, and sent the patient to the surgical intensive care unit. Just then, Steinberg came in. "Where were you?" demanded Dr. Islam. "At home; where do you think? I'm not on call," replied Dr. Steinberg. Are there any ethical issues involved in this situation? How should such situations be handled?

FEMINIST ETHICS

Although virtue ethics is historically ancient, the approach is just now being applied to professional ethics, which, generally, has been treated as a series of isolated problems rather than an expression of how to live a good life. Part of the impetus to examine virtue ethics comes from the recognition that, for professionals, careers are inextricable parts of our lives—of who we are—and not merely a series of problems to solve or activities to perform. Similarly, although women's involvement in health care is ancient and women have historically influenced the values of the health care professions, it is only fairly recently that feminist philosophers and scholars have begun to think carefully about the ways in which the traditional feminization of health care apart from medical specialties influences or ought to influence our understanding of ethical values in professional practice.

An example is the health professions' traditional ethic of care, or caring. Carol Gilligan (1982) used these terms to describe an ethic that "cannot be 'laced up in formulas'"—as she says, moral judgment cannot be bound by "general rules" but must instead be informed "by a life vivid and intense enough to have created a wide fellow-feeling with all that is human" (p. 130). And while this may not be all of what nursing, for example, means by "caring," her point that an adequate ethic cannot be merely a matter of honoring principles or calculating outcomes is surely right.

Another perspective on the relationship between an ethic of care and other theories is this:

> Whereas equity is directed toward the welfare of society as a whole, based on abstract principles of fairness, care is concerned with the welfare of people without necessary regard for fairness. Whereas equity emphasizes fair procedures, care insists on benevolence and kindness. Equity asks that we do our duty in accordance with reason, but care insists that we act out of concern. While equity may be administered blindly—the image of Justice, blindfolded, holding her scales, is apt—care can only be given by a human face. While equity asks that we act out of a sense of self-interest as well as the interests of others, care focuses on the interests of others. (Oliner and Oliner, 1998)

The emphasis in this passage on caring and relationship as valid elements of a responsible ethic is related to the work of feminist and feminist-influenced ethicists in recent years. Feminism is not one phenomenon, and feminist ethics is not one idea about ethics. Rather, each is a tradition undergoing continued development. Nevertheless, it may be helpful to identify certain themes within this tradition that characterize it as a distinct stream of thought.

In general, feminist thinkers draw attention to ways in which women find themselves and their concerns subordinated to those of men in virtually all the ways that matter to them and others—in the spheres of political, social, and economic power as well as in interpersonal relationships and their internal dynamics. Two kinds of responses to that subordination can be seen as having particular importance in feminist writing. One is to challenge it in every morally acceptable way as unjustifiable oppression and attempt to recast social, political, economic, and other relationships in ways that promote genuinely mutual respect and equality. The other is to draw attention to the unique contributions traditionally feminine values—such as caring and sensitivity to relationship—can make to a more adequate ethic and to promote those values as counterweights to traditionally masculine patterns of ethical reasoning that emphasize impersonal justice or consequentialist considerations. Of course, these two kinds of responses are not mutually exclusive; in the work of many feminist writers—and the lives of many people— they are intimately bound together in theory and practice. In order to explore these perspectives further, consider this case.

Case 6.5: Feminist Ethics and Workplace Harassment

From the perspective of Community Hospital, Dr. Patel is nearly a model physician: he brings in lots of patients, performs his administrative work conscientiously, and offers skilled and attentive care to his patients. To nurses and support staff, however, Dr. Patel is arrogant and demeaning, seldom missing an opportunity to criticize what he feels is inadequate performance. What really infuriates Dr. Patel most, however, is the slightest failure to show him what he feels is proper deference. Questioning his orders, even for purposes of clarification, is met with withering sarcasm; offering one's own observations provokes degrading personal remarks.

Amanda R. is a case manager working with Mr. Abrams, Dr. Patel's patient, and it is quite clear to her, as well as to the nurses who have worked with him, that Mr. Abrams would benefit from home-care nursing visits and occupational therapy. Dr. Patel, however, has not answered Amanda's four telephone calls and brusquely shoved past her when she attempted to speak with him in the hall. Finally, Amanda spoke with Mr. Abrams's family, who, at her urging, went to Dr. Patel's office and demanded that he order the care Amanda and the nurses had recommended. He acquiesced in this, but, as soon as they had left, Dr. Patel subjected Amanda to a blistering tirade over the telephone, ending with his promise to get Amanda fired if she ever so much as thought about pulling another end run around his orders. In tears, Amanda went home early and thought hard about resigning.

Has Dr. Patel behaved unethically in this situation? One does not have to analyze this case from a specifically feminist perspective to see that his actions are clearly cruel and offensive, but bringing out exactly how his actions are professionally unethical in terms of violations of principles or consequentialist calculations can be difficult and may not capture the true depth of his wrongdoing. However, from both the feminist perspectives mentioned above, that emphasing the wrongness of oppressive subordination and that emphasizing the importance of caring relationship, what is wrong with Dr. Patel's behavior is clear. He is perpetuating an old, stereotypical, male-dominant kind of behavior in which a subordinate professional position is demeaned, as if those who hold such positions are somehow inferior human beings, unworthy of collegial respect or even recognition of their dignity as people. Moreover, the kind of relationship he insists on here is devoid of trust, with no concern for or interest in those he considers his inferiors; it offers them no opportunity to collaborate on anything like professional terms and exploits them for an unacceptably narrow range of purposes, principally to massage Dr. Patel's ego.

It is certainly unreasonable to suggest that health care delivery can dispense with working relationships in which some members of the health care team work under the orders of others or in which their roles are actually subordinate to others. Differences in responsibility, legal obligations, education, authority, and other matters mandate differences in role relationships because they assure better and more efficient delivery of care. However, nothing in the relationship of subordination needs to entail diminished respect for people as colleagues or license oppressive or degrading treatment of subordinates by others. The model toward which health care is moving, and ought to be moving, is one in which health care providers collaborate respectfully with each other, benefiting clients through the full deployment of everyone's expertise. A multiplicity of educational backgrounds and professional and personal perspectives provides the best possible environment to assure that no important needs or values at stake in any situation are simply ignored. Behavior like Dr. Patel's not only is counterproductive of such a collaborative model of care but also actually threatens client care by assigning to only one person, the physician alone, all the expertise and understanding necessary to practice effectively—while alienating other members of the health care team whose cooperation is important for the most successful outcome.

Gilligan (1982) and Noddings (1984) have each argued that one characteristically feminine way of dealing with value conflicts is to do in any particular situation what preserves relationship while expressing caring interest. In relationships that express caring, concrete interactions between particular people that advance the "cared-for's" interests do not, at the same time, cost the "carer" unreasonably and certainly do not strip her of her dignity. Instead, appropriately caring relationships have five characteristics. They fulfill the one doing the caring; they call on the unique and particular individuality of the one doing the caring; they are not produced by a person in a role because of gender, with one gender engaging in nurturing behavior and the other engaging in instrumental (using, taking advantage) behavior; they are reciprocated with caring, and not merely with the satisfaction of seeing the ones cared for flourishing and pursuing other projects; and finally, they take place within a framework of consciousness-raising practice and conversation.[3]

Clearly, however, Dr. Patel's behavior makes this sort of relationship impossible. Bullying and disregarding the professionally responsible contributions of his colleagues makes it impossible for them to find fulfillment in their work while denying them any uniqueness or individuality. It is precisely Dr. Patel's expectation that his colleagues are merely to be used for his own purposes, not cared about and respected as people, that is so offensive. And clearly his intimidating threats of reprisals create the sort of hostile environment in which oppressive practices cannot be addressed.

The problem for Amanda and others similarly victimized by this sort of oppression is finding a way to deal with the problem that is not unreasonably risky and promises some improvement. Most informal means to deal with people like Dr. Patel—social ostracism, working to the exact letter of one's responsibilities but providing no more than the bare minimum necessary to avoid disciplinary action, and the like—are either unlikely to be effective or will threaten patient welfare, or both.

Fortunately, however, it is becoming increasingly common for victimized subordinates to have recourse to complaints of harassment, "creating a hostile work environment," and the like, which, when appropriately documented, can lead to disciplinary action including suspension of practice privileges or dismissal. Where institutions have interests vested in a physician's ability to bring in patients or other political and economic issues are relevant, it can be difficult to induce the appropriate supervisors or administrators to act. However, the increasing seriousness with which sexual harassment cases are being taken is helping to create pressure not to disregard concerns of similar seriousness that are not specifically sexual.

---

[3] Sheila Mullet, "Shifting Perspectives: A New Approach to Ethics," in Lorraine Code, Sheila Mullett, and Christine Overall, eds., *Feminist Perspectives* (Toronto: University of Toronto, 1989), pp. 119–120. We have made slight changes for clarity.

Have you met people like Dr. Patel? How have you dealt with people like
him? If you were in Amanda's place, how would you handle her situation?

Many ethicists and health care practitioners would credit feminism with important contributions toward a more humane world as well as one in which important but neglected concerns, especially of women, are increasingly being taken seriously. Feminist ethicists are not without their critics, however. Among the more serious charges against them are that their ideas lead to a kind of reverse sexism and stereotyping in which feminine virtues are touted as superior to masculine virtues—charges that a "gendered" approach to ethics is necessarily sexist. While it may be true that principled and consequentialist considerations do not provide a sufficiently rich conception of ethics—or provide one that does not do justice to women's experiences—those perspectives are not at all unimportant and, as a practical matter, profoundly influence ethical reasoning and ought to do so. It is also arguable that strident feminist criticism can alienate people who would otherwise be supportive, degrade choices that many women find fulfilling, and undermine effective working relationships.

But none of these criticisms needs to be especially compelling. If feminist ethics does not "systematically exclude the interests, identities, issues, and values of one or the other of the two sexes" or lose sight of the fact that men as much as women can express care and resist oppressive human relationships, ethical awareness of gender need not be considered sexist (Tong, 1997, p. 92). If feminist ethics does not propose to banish considerations of justice and attention to consequences from ethical discussion, but rather to insist on the importance of other values, too, that need hardly be treated as an attack on principled and consequentialist reasoning. And feminist criticism need not be strident and divisive, judgmental and alienating any more than any other ethical perspective is. On the contrary, if the goal is to get a sympathetic hearing from people whose perspectives vary greatly, patient, persistent goodwill seems a much more plausible strategy, at least in general.

THE "CONTINUUM OF ETHICAL
DECISION MAKING" AGAIN

We have now studied a number of ethical dead ends, as well as four perspectives that offer certain important advantages and some disadvantages. While many people earnestly wish for a single ethical decision procedure and not all philosophers or moralists have given up hope for one, we believe that the immense diversity of human interests and concerns; the diversity of cultures, traditions, and ways of thinking; and widely differing circumstances make this unlikely. Instead, what we have been suggesting is that each of these approaches—reasoning from consequences, reasoning from principles, reasoning from professionalism, and the practice of virtue or character—enriched with a deeper appreciation of feminist perspectives and combined with a considerable body of shared deep values and a willingness to reason patiently and sympathetically, giving due attention to the best information available, can offer the best possibility of resolving conflicts in ethically acceptable ways. Nyberg (1993) puts a similar point this way:

> If collisions of value are unavoidable, if only some but not all conflicting values can live easily together, if human lives can be fashioned and lived imaginatively only in a pattern of mutually exclusive choices, then what can we do? The answer is: make adjustments as best we can, to avoid extremes of suffering and soften the blows. . . . A history of conventions, attachments to particular people and institutions, commitment, a sense of character or integrity—all of these go into a moral point of view, along with whatever guidance reason, rules, principles can provide. In the end, if anything binds us to moral conduct of a certain kind it cannot be only principles or rules. More likely it will be a sense not wholly understood, an intuition that this is the right thing to do, all things considered. We may not do the best thing we can imagine doing, but it will be the best we can manage in the circumstances. (p. 199ff.)

Our suggestion is that a judicious combination of sensitivities to principles, consequences, and character can help us understand how to know what is the best thing we can do, as well as to help others share and accept our understanding.

QUESTIONS FOR DISCUSSION

1. A number of recent writers, including Carol Gilligan and Nel Noddings, have argued that women in general may be less likely than men in general to approach ethical decision making from perspectives like consequentialism or principled reasoning. Instead, they suggest, many women are more likely to approach each situation from a perspective of caring, in which preservation or development of relationship is seen as a primary value. If Ann were to approach case 6.1 from this perspective, how do you think she would handle Sandy's case? Would such an approach be ethically responsible? Why or why not?

2. Suppose you were asked to rank-order the following list of virtues from the point of view of a health care employer: professional competence, cooperation, integrity, friendliness, compassion for others, tact, industry (being a hard worker), punctuality, and

assertiveness. Which do you think are the most important in a potential employee? Which are the least? Why?

3. Some feminist writers emphasize that typical health care environments often function in ways that consistently neglect, downplay, trivialize, or simply pay no attention to women practitioners or their concerns, insights, or perspectives. Do you think this claim is true? What specific examples can you cite to substantiate it? If it is true, how can women get their concerns a more respected hearing?

PART III

Health Care Issues for Discussion

In this section of the text, four important issues with public policy implications will be introduced. These issues are the "crisis" in health care and health care reform (Chapter 7), the ethics of euthanasia, physician-assisted suicide, and end-of-life decisions (Chapter 8), ethical issues and genetic research (Chapter 9), and confidentiality in health care in the Information Age (Chapter 10).

In various ways, all of these issues loom prominently in health care policy discussions while, at the same time, personally affect most health care professionals at one time or another, in their professional capacities, as private citizens, and as recipients of health care. In democratic societies, we place a great premium on resolving issues of public policy by developing some sort of consensus through informed debate. We believe that it is essential for health care professionals to participate actively in the debates surrounding these issues because, if they do not, the discussion is likely to be preempted by groups far less knowledgeable about the realities of health care and guided far more by narrow self-interest and counterproductive ideologies.

That is not to say that health care professionals will necessarily speak with one voice on the issues we will be discussing. And, though we try, we cannot claim that our discussion of these issues is absolutely evenhanded. After all, even the idea that public policy issues ought to be resolved by educated discussion and consensus building among competing pluralistic viewpoints is itself an idea that not everyone in our society currently accepts. Moreover, these issues are not quietly sitting on the sidelines awaiting rational discussion; they are being debated loud and long right now. So our presentation of the issues here should be regarded only as a beginning point for further discussion. Because of the evolving nature of the discussion of these issues, we expect that some of our ideas may be "old" by the time you read them. As a result of this evolution, you will have a larger pool of ideas and commentary for your discussion and presentation of these issues. But, we suspect, the issues we have chosen here, like the controversies surrounding abortion, are unlikely to be resolved to everyone's satisfaction anytime soon because they each involve conflicts among powerful values with passionate constituencies.

Our goal in this section of the text is to explain what the most important of these conflicts, values, and constituencies probably are in a way that encourages people to think about them carefully and to arrive at their own ethically justifiable conclusions. That is, once more, we encourage people to follow the method we have advocated throughout the earlier sections of this book, beginning with fact-finding, and proceeding to identifying the most important values at stake in each situation, and so on to a defensible conclusion. Fact-finding is especially important in these issues for two reasons. First, in the public policy arena, the facts, and especially how the facts are interpreted, change rapidly, so current information is crucial. And, second, unfortunately, much of the debate over these health care issues is not securely based on any facts; all too often, it is based on untested assumptions and impassioned political rhetoric. It is therefore all the more necessary to pursue all the information that is relevant to a rational decision, at least if any real progress is to be made toward a resolution.

CHAPTER SEVEN

The American Health Care Crisis

ACCESS TO HEALTH CARE

Critics of the American health care system characterize its current condition as a crisis. Whether this is a fair description and how alarming the situation is depend on people's individual circumstances, as well as how much credence they give to statistics provided by the government and other sources. Almost everyone seems to know horrific anecdotes about malpractice and neglect, catastrophic expenses, and appallingly callous treatment, yet there also seems to be an abundance of miraculous cures, lives saved and restored to health and well-being. What, then, is the problem?

Case 7.1: Living Without Health Care Insurance

John and Maria G. married two years out of high school. While John was employed full-time mounting and spin-balancing tires at Discount Tire Mart and Maria worked at Classy Cuts Salon, they were able to rent a small house for $400 a month and otherwise get by reasonably well, even though neither of their employers offered health insurance or other benefits. Last year, however, Maria became pregnant due to contraceptive failure. Strongly opposed to abortion, both John and Maria decided they would have their baby, conscientiously making use of low-cost prenatal care available through a local clinic. But that subsidized health care is no longer available, and Maria has had to quit her job to care for their daughter. So the family is now living on John's minimum-wage income alone, which is approximately $10,500 a year. Concerned about providing adequate health care for his family, John contacted a local insurance agent about a "bare bones" policy. With a $250 yearly deductible, John was quoted a premium of $3,500 a year, or 35 percent of their annual income.

Case 7.2: Health Care Options with Insurance

Diane B. teaches biology at John Glenn High School. Her union contract offers Diane three health care choices: traditional Blue Cross/Blue Shield comprehensive coverage at a $20 premium each pay-period, "K-Care," an HMO associated with a major regional health center with an office a few blocks from Diane's suburban home, or Health Plus, a preferred provider organization. Both of the latter are available to Diane without cost; she became a member of the HMO because of cost, convenience, and a good relationship with her primary physician. Diane recently suffered persist-ent pain in the middle right area of her chest. After an ultrasound and a CT scan revealed some anomalies in the area of her pancreas, she had an endoscopic retrograde cholepancreatography (a fiber-optic examination), which revealed some pancreatitis. After taking a mild acid blocker and following her physician's advice about some lifestyle changes, a follow-up CT scan six weeks later revealed that the pancreatitis had largely cleared up and the previous anomalies had nearly disappeared.

It is estimated that approximately 40 million Americans, like John, Maria, and their daughter, lack health insurance. This number is growing rapidly: up 50 percent in the past 15 years by some estimates. Medicare cov-ers all but 0.3 percent of America's seniors (along with 5 million Americans under 65 who are either disabled or in end-stage renal disease). However, 68 percent of seniors also purchase supplemental policies to extend or add benefits not otherwise covered (such as eye care, outpatient prescriptions, preventive care, and psychological care). Eligibility for nursing home care requires depletion of all but $2,000 in assets. But Medicare is in serious financial trouble. In June 1996, Rep. Bill Archer, chairman of the House Ways and Means Committee, predicted that Medicare will have an $86 bil-lion deficit by 2002, rather than the $5 billion surplus trustees predicted only one year earlier. Medicaid covers 25 million low-income mothers and children (most of whom also receive some form of aid to dependent chil-dren), as well as some blind and disabled patients. However, Medicaid nor-mally reimburses only 60–80 percent of costs for primary care, so only 6 percent of the budget goes to those physicians who will see such patients. Forty percent of those below the poverty line are covered by Medicaid. The rest, like John and Maria, are uninsured. And, like Medicare, Medicaid is under serious reexamination due to extravagant increases in costs.

Now, suppose that Maria had experienced the chest pain, rather than Diane. Diane's treatment was billed at approximately $6,200; but, because of her excellent benefits, Diane paid nothing out of pocket. However, if her treatment had been paid out of pocket, it would proba-bly have been billed at a higher rate. Because her HMO is associated with a regional medical center, the medical center's charges for ultrasound and CT scan services are 27 percent lower; because the ERCP was performed there by a physician under contract to the center, it too was billed at about 75 percent of the normal rate. If Maria had been treated as Diane was, she and John would have been facing a bill in the neighborhood of $8,300. Remember, their annual income is approximately $10,500; and bear in mind that, after rent and taxes, the family is trying to live on $3,600 a year ($300 a month for food, utilities, clothing, transportation, health care, and all the other incidental expenses of living). It is obvious that Maria will not be able to receive the kind of treatment that Diane did.

What would Maria do if she had the same symptoms as Diane? Probably she would simply ignore the pain as long as she could. And if its cause was a pancreas inflamed by temporary lifestyle changes, it is probable that the problem would resolve itself. But Maria would not likely interpret her symptoms as episodic pancreatitis. More likely, Maria would think that her symptoms were a gallbladder problem, or cancer, or even, depending on her level of health education, a heart attack. And any of those things would be possible so far as anyone would know before examination (remember, Diane's problem was identified only after a battery of tests). When the pain became intolerable, more than likely Maria would present herself at the medical center's emergency room. There, the care Maria would receive, depending on diagnostic studies performed, would cost two to three times what it would if it were done on an outpatient basis.

Once she arrived at the emergency room, Maria's experience would vary greatly depending on the policies of the medical center. If the medical center were a private institution, Maria would quite possibly be turned away, though it would normally be determined that she was stable before she would be referred elsewhere. Because she is indigent, uninsured, and without Medicaid, the medical center would have almost no chance to make up its costs. Rather than incur these unreimbursed costs, medical center policies would probably require sending Maria to a public hospital. An increasing number of private medical centers will not take a case like Maria's even if the patient has Medicaid, because current levels of reimbursement range between 60 and 75 percent of customary billings, which does not even begin to meet the hospitals' costs.

In 1998, Congress's attempt to deal with spiraling Medicaid costs resulted in actual reductions by pushing down reimbursement levels even further. One Midwest medical center received $5,000,000 less in fiscal year 1999 for the same number of Medicaid patients served as a result of this new initiative: same number of patients, same level of care, just $5,000,000 less.

But public hospitals are no better off; in fact, by many measures they are much worse off. For example, of 277 public hospitals in one survey, 47 percent have turned away uninsured patients. Of 250,000 emergency room visits in Los Angeles in one year, 40 percent had neither insurance nor Medicare or Medicaid. Because nonprofit public hospitals are having to absorb enormous unreimbursed costs and the rest of their case loads are increasingly being made up of Medicaid/ Medicare patients, remaining financially viable is extraordinarily difficult. To remain solvent, public hospitals have to compete with private medical centers for those patients, like Diane, whose private insurance is more generous; they hope to recoup some of their losses by "cost shifting." That is, in effect, they will overcharge Diane's insurer to make up for the losses suffered on Maria, as well as Medicare and Medicaid patients. So, for example, a typical nonurgent emergency room visit costing $62 may be billed at $125 to $150; meanwhile, markup on supplies is frequently between 75 percent and 85 percent. While some of this money goes to recover losses from uncompensated care, much of it is also directed to basic operating costs such as medical center utility expenses and staff salaries.

Diane's HMO is unlikely to go along with this practice, and neither are other major private health insurance companies. In fact, when Medicare and Medicaid began to reimburse care based on diagnostic related groups (DRGs) in 1983, many insurers began to restrict their reimbursement to amounts approved under these same DRGs.

DRG (diagnostic related group) reimbursement *provides a geographically set rate of reimbursement for a host of diagnoses based on average costs for treatment. In effect, a health care facility is given a fixed amount of reimbursement for providing required inpatient care no matter what the actual costs for that care were.*

Reimbursement by DRGs was intended to encourage efficiencies by providing financial incentives for quick, effective treatment. Reimbursement by DRGs did reduce lengths of stays and reduce costs, at least initially. However, this approach also winds up rewarding institutions whose client populations are relatively healthy and penalizing those whose client load is relatively sicker. Moreover, by holding down DRG reimbursement levels, third-party payers have created other problems. Some patients are being prematurely discharged and inadequately treated, while those who remain in hospitals are *much* sicker. The DRG reimbursement system also influences the shift of care from the inpatient arena to the outpatient arena because it is cheaper. Same-day surgery for formerly inpatient procedures is the result of this shift. However, most health care facilities are now preparing for a similar reimbursement system for outpatient care that is expected to be implemented in 2000.

According to the Government Accounting Office (GAO), $17 billion a year is lost due to fraudulent billing practices: billing for a heart bypass operation but actually performing an angioplasty, for example. Such fraud is not necessarily due merely to greed: it can also be due to efforts to recoup otherwise unreimbursed charges. In spite of these efforts, 57 percent of hospitals were on the loss side of DRG reimbursements in 1994. In 1990, public hospitals in Philadelphia alone lost $85 million. The only remaining hospital in East St. Louis has now closed, along with 17 hospitals in the Chicago area; similar statistics can be found virtually throughout the country.

Billing for care is a complex activity requiring the utilization of thousands of codes assigned to specific disease entities and procedures. Most health care providers are dependent on highly skilled medical records personnel to perform this activity-based documentation in the patient's medical record.

Another by-product of these efforts to contain costs is a boom in home health care. Since 1984, home health care has increased 275 percent, providing 6 percent of all health care services. Home health care is normally cost-effective, especially in comparison to hospitalization: $531 a day for home care versus $2,263 a day in a hospital is a customary ratio; the GAO estimates that Medicare saves $575 million annually because of home care. But home care brings problems as well as benefits. Loads can be heavy: 18 home visits a day is an average load for a home-care nurse (an 18-patient-a-day case load for one nurse means 26.6 minutes maximum for each patient including travel time); there is little collegial support or backup for problem cases; quality of care provided is largely unsupervised; fraud is not uncommon; and great discrepancies exist in pricing for services.

But the uninsured are unlikely to receive home care because they can't afford it. Maria and other uninsured patients are unlikely to pursue treatments for any conditions that are not acute and episodic. So, for example, she is almost certain to forgo occupational or physical therapy unless she is incapacitated, and then she is likely to participate only until she can cope with the most necessary demands of daily living. She is unlikely to fill prescriptions she thinks she can do without. And she is unlikely to seek adequate dental or vision care, not to mention psychological care. Even if Maria were a Medicaid patient, there would be powerful disincentives for individual providers, just like hospitals, to treat her.

Table 7.1   Comparison of Physician Salaries—1996 Figures

All physicians' mean net income	$199,000, up 1.8% from 1995
Radiology	$275,000, up 12.6% from 1995
Surgery	$275,000, up 2.2% from 1995
Anesthesiology	$228,400, up 6.2% from 1995
General practice/family practice	$139,100, up 6.0% from 1995

Source: Bloom (1998).

Case 7.3: Conscientious Practice Versus Low Reimbursement Levels

Laura C., D.O., was recruited to a group practice in a county with only one major community of about 25,000 and an otherwise rural environment. As usual in such arrangements, Laura was promised a minimum salary by the group for a period of three years, after which she would receive a share determined by the group's revenues and her client load. Laura is every patient's dream for a family practitioner. She devotes extra time to those who need it; she is willing to listen patiently, even when her patient load is high, to hear what her clients want to say. She explains problems and treatments thoroughly; and she is highly regarded and much loved by her patients, especially young mothers and the elderly, as the result. While her patients and their families love her, physician members of her group are dissatisfied with her performance. Because Laura is willing to care for many Medicare/Medicaid patients and spends so much time with her patients, her financial contribution to the group is much lower than that of her peers. In effect, her conscientiousness and caring is reducing the entire group's revenues. Most of her colleagues are seeing nearly twice the number of patients Laura sees and they also limit the number of Medicare/Medicaid patients to less than 20 percent of their load. Her colleagues are now urging Laura to do the same or face a significant reduction in her income. This places Laura in an uncomfortable professional dilemma. She has to decide if she should reduce the time she spends with her patients, accept a reduction of income, or perhaps risk losing her job.

Of course, some would argue that physician income is a significant part of the problem. In 1993, a *Newsweek* poll reported that 83 percent of Americans believed that physicians charge too much. And regardless of the public's impression, it seems clear that American physicians are comparatively well paid, as Table 7.1 reveals.

These income figures are means; furthermore, unlike those in most other nations, most American physicians (70 percent) are specialists

Table 7.2   *Overview of Some Unnecessary Operations*

Procedure	Appropriate: need based on patient condition—%	Equivocal: need probable based on patient condition—%	Inappropriate: not needed based on patient condition—%
Coronary angiography	74	9	17
Coronary artery bypasses	56	30	14
Pacemaker insert	44	36	20
Carotid endarterectomy	36	32	32
Endoscopy	72	11	17

Source: Brooks (1990).

rather than general practitioners. Moreover, although $199,000 looks like a lot of money from the standpoint of the average American wage, it is comparable to the income of some other highly educated professionals and corporate leaders, most of whom don't have the costs incurred by physicians in the course of their practices or much of the personal responsibility that generates malpractice complaints and lawsuits. Yet in countries where health care is regarded as a public service and physicians are employees of governments, physician salaries are comparable to those of other government employees, such as university professors and judges, rather than to salaries of the best-paid members of the private sector.

Quite apart from whether American physicians are too well paid, it is often thought that physicians, practicing defensive medicine and unconcerned about costs, order unneeded tests and perform unnecessary procedures. And there is some evidence to support these claims (Table 7.2).

Other sources have speculated that 20–50 percent of commonly performed specialty procedures could have been avoided without harming public health. And one might argue that at least one of the CT scans or the endoscopy that Diane underwent for pancreatitis was superfluous. Yet physicians argue that hindsight is always a better predictor of whether a procedure is necessary than the best estimate prior to that procedure.

Authorization by the insurer for a procedure is required for reimbursement for the procedure. Many third-party payers now require a second opinion from a physician of their choice for procedures before this authorization is given.

Even though many physicians may not know the cost of tests or procedures they prescribe (or even, sometimes, the cost of their own office

Table 7.3   The Uninsured by Income Level

Annual Income	Uninsured Non-Elderly Population
Less than $5,000	4,400,000
$5,000 to $9,999	5,100,000
$10,000 to $14,999	5,600,000
$15,000 to $19,999	4,700,000
$20,000 to $29,999	6,600,000
$30,000 to $39,999	3,800,000
$40,000 to $49,999	2,400,000
$50,000 and over	3,800,000
Total	36,300,000

visits), it is doubtful that the quality of American health care would be improved if physicians constantly balanced considerations of cost-effectiveness against the prices of therapies. This, in fact, is one principal objection to HMOs: that their treatments are based on cost-effectiveness rather than conscientious care.

Current debates about health care reform tend to focus on two issues: increasing access to health care and restraining growth in health care costs, especially where Medicare and Medicaid are concerned. As we have seen in the case of John and Maria, given that people working a 40-hour week, 50 weeks a year, at the current minimum wage are making about $10,500 before taxes and given the costs of housing, food, clothing, and other necessities, it is not difficult to understand why the working poor are generally uninsured.

In fact, it is not difficult to understand why many people, about 13 percent of the population, go uninsured unless their employers or a public agency provide insurance for them. Table 7.3 reveals that being uninsured is not merely a question of total income.

Eighty-five percent of the uninsured are employed or dependents of people who are employed. By occupation, 40 percent of agricultural workers, 35 percent in personal services, 31 percent in construction, 26 percent in business and repair services, 25 percent in retail, 22 percent of the self-employed outside of agriculture, and 20 percent of people employed in recreation and entertainment are uninsured. They are disproportionately young, minority, and male, and live in the South and West, although 16 million women and 27.1 million nonminorities are uninsured. The upshot is that the public school teacher with tennis elbow is likely to be able to get a $1,000 MRI (magnetic resonance imaging) scan at little or no cost to himself, but a waitress earning minimum wage may find it impossible to pay $60 for the mammogram that could save her life.

In 1990, a typical poor uninsured adult like Maria saw or spoke with a physician about four times over the course of the year compared with six contacts for an equally poor adult who did have private insurance. The uninsured are also less able to provide health care for their children. Preschool children covered by Medicaid had 6.0 physician visits in 1990 while uninsured children averaged 2.8 visits. And only 55 percent of those visits were to a doctor's office, as compared to 78 percent for insured children. Instead, uninsured children are seen in emergency rooms, hospital outpatient departments, and clinics, where expenses are dramatically higher. As we have seen, many of these expenses cannot be recovered.

What values are at stake in this situation? At first sight, the American health care system lacks fairness. There is a kind of social Darwinist element in the system, in that it rewards the more socially productive (or well-employed) members but not those who are less successful. The criteria of success in this calculation are those characteristic of materialistic, market-driven societies like ours. So our health care system distributes benefits to the affluent, who can pay for them themselves, and to the well-insured, who are most often members of well-educated or politically powerful groups. But such a practice utterly overlooks the importance of the interests of the more than 40 million Americans who are not well served by our system.

> One of our American values is market justice—the idea that if a person can afford something, he or she has the "right," through purchase, to have it. Extended to health care, this idea or value implies that health care is a commodity like any other and that people such as the poor and underinsured have no more right or entitlement to health care than they have to any other product they cannot afford. "Market justice" is one way of allocating—or rationing—health care services, but critics question how just it really is.

It is reasonably common to consider adequate access to health care a human right; the United Nations Declaration of the Rights of Man, to which the United States is a signatory, asserts this, as do many professional codes of ethics in health care fields. Without making heavy use of this concept of rights, it still seems reasonable to say that there is something ethically problematic about a society such as ours that purports to value equality and fairness, that is the richest economy in the world, and that nevertheless effectively disenfranchises a substantial portion of its population from one of the most essential of human goods.

If we take seriously the idea that society has a moral obligation to assure access to health care, it is vitally important to ask about the extent and nature of this obligation. No matter how wealthy our society may be, we have only limited resources to meet health care needs that can be virtually limitless. Here, conceptual issues leap out immediately. If universal or at least much-expanded access to health care is an ethical obligation, it seems reasonable that we know or have a common understanding of what is meant by "health." The American medical system tends to define health as the absence of disease, a definition that is both unhelpful conceptually (what makes something a disease?) and restrictive in practice (because it turns physicians into disease-care providers). Some theorists offer a concept of health that is more inclusive and at the same time relativistic. For example, "Health transcends biological fitness. It is primarily a measure of each person's ability to do what he wants to do and become what he wants to become" (Dubos, 1961). The World Health Organization defines health even more expansively as a "state of complete well-being, physical, social, and mental, and not merely the absence of disease or infirmity" (cited in Deloughery, 1991). Surely these definitions are right in stressing that health is more than a condition of being disease-free. But they are also profoundly problematic.

If people have a right to health, and health is defined in Dubos's terms—enabling people to do what they want—do we have an obligation to promote someone's desire to smoke, drink to excess, or abuse drugs? If we adopt a definition as expansive as that of the World Health Organization, is there any limit to what a right to health might entitle people to have? Quite apart from what it might take to provide complete well-being in spheres other than the physical, should society even ensure that everyone who needs and wants *any and all* sophisticated or exotic therapies should have access to them? This idea of health care as a right is not only impossible as a practical matter because of cost and resource availability issues (there is neither enough money nor enough donor organ availability to provide everyone who wants one with a medically warranted transplant, for example). It is also unwise as an ideal, because it substitutes limitless consumption for personal responsibility.

Risky behavior is not just bungee-cord jumping and skydiving. Risky behavior also includes driving without a seat belt, riding a motorcycle without a helmet, and snowmobiling under the influence of alcohol. If risky behavior involves actions that place us at greater risk for health problems, then failure to have yearly Pap examinations or dental checkups could also be considered risky behavior. Do we want to go this far?

But, if limitless access to any and all procedures is not a possible goal (and it's not), the process of drawing lines becomes inevitable, as do questions about where lines should be drawn. Make no mistake: lines are being drawn now, but mostly invisibly. Typically healthy, wealthy, and politically powerful individuals and groups are imposing policy decisions on the sick, poor, and politically weak. These policy decisions are not usually crafted by the kind of ethical decision-making procedure we have been working with. Many of them are not even made as elements of a deliberate health care policy. Yet, collectively, decisions by individual care providers, insurance company employees, public health officials, and government leaders have had the effect of excluding 40 million Americans from access to our system and millions more from access to the best care our system has to offer.

From an ethical perspective, it seems obvious that lines should be drawn fairly, or justly, rather than arbitrarily. Minimally, this means that unless there are relevant differences between them, similar cases should be treated similarly. Currently, lines are drawn on the basis of wealth: those who have it can have any procedure they want or need. Those who lack wealth may lack access to even the most rudimentary health care. So, unless one thinks wealth is relevant to whether one deserves access to health care, the current system is unjust and unfair.

If wealth is not relevant or is not the only relevant consideration in allocating health care, what is relevant? People in rural areas obviously have less access to health care than some people in suburban areas based on the place of their residence. The same is true of people in inner-city neighborhoods. Should access be equalized regardless of geography? How could it be achieved? Women characteristically use 25 percent more medical care than men. The elderly characteristically use about 33 percent more than nonelderly patients. Should we put 25–33 percent more resources into women's and elderly health services? Or should women and the elderly constitute a separate risk pool that is billed at rates 25–33 percent higher?

Should considerations of individual responsibility influence allocation decisions? A famous article asks "Who Should Pay for Smokers' Medical Care?" (Veatch, 1974), and an increasingly popular answer among society and insurance companies is "smokers themselves." Carrying this theme beyond the currently unfashionable smoker, should *all* health problems attributable to voluntary risk behavior be the financial responsibility of those who engage in it? "You play, you pay" then becomes the rule for motorcyclists, skiers, and hang gliders. But what about other risks? For example, people who keep guns in their houses are much more likely to require medical attention than those who do not. People who eat junk food, or eggs and bacon for breakfast more than twice a week, or fish from some parts of the Great Lakes—or who drink large amounts of cola, coffee, or whiskey—are all voluntarily increasing their risks. So are those who weigh more than 10 percent over the ideal weight for their height. And, of course, those who have children radically increase the burden on society's health care budget because of the greater health care needs of children. Should all these risk-increasing actions disqualify people from socially guaranteed health care?

Should lines be drawn on the basis of assuring everyone access to certain procedures, while access to other procedures would be limited to those who could afford them on their own? This is in effect what the Oregon health care rationing plan does: through public debate, a prioritized list of procedures is developed, and the state pays for as many of them as it can given its health care budget. Anything else is the responsibility of individual patients. But is this fair to victims of less common or stigmatized diseases or conditions (such as AIDS or schizophrenia)?

We can multiply questions about health policy indefinitely. The purpose of this section, however, is only to draw attention to ethical issues related to cost and access in the American health care system. Assuming that the existence of serious ethical issues cannot reasonably be denied or ignored, the next problem is to develop social policies and the political will to implement health care reform. We would hope that such policies would be developed through a process of thoughtful, democratic deliberation in which health care professionals would be prepared to take a leading role. In the next section, we examine some of the public policy initiatives and ideas that have attracted at least some support among health policy advocates.

QUESTIONS FOR DISCUSSION

1. *Case 7.4: Preferential Treatment in the Waiting Room*—While attending a weeklong conference at a large urban university located in the inner city, Jane S., who is the director of physical plant and sterile processing services at a suburban, public hospital in another state, has experienced several increasingly painful bouts of gastrointestinal pain. On entering the triage area of the inner-city hospital nearest the university, she encounters a room full of people: wailing children, distraught mothers, addicts experiencing withdrawal symptoms, people with injuries wrapped in towels and rags, virtually all of whom are either black or Hispanic. (Jane is a non-Hispanic white.) Surprisingly, the admitting nurse approached Jane after only a few minutes, took her information (including her private insurance provider's card), and promptly ushered her into an examining room. While waiting for the harassed young resident who joined her in a few minutes, Jane

observed that the room was a mess: huge "dust bunnies," blood, and other unidentifiable matter were on the floor; the examining table had no paper covering, only ancient, creased plastic; and the cabinets, whose doors were open, looked empty. The resident ruefully acknowledged that even minimal standards of asepsis were not being met, but pointed out that, with only himself and two nurses on duty, they could *either* clean rooms *or* see patients; and with the incredible backlog outside, it seemed to him that seeing patients had better be the priority. What do you see as the most ethically troubling aspects of this case? What do you think accounts for the situation described above? What reasonably should be done to turn this situation around?

2. Put yourself in the position of John and Maria, whose case appeared at the beginning of this chapter. How would you reply to someone who argued that there is nothing truly unfair or unjust in their situation and that their mistake was simply failing to abort the child they could not afford? (Make sure the ethical basis of your response is clearly articulated.)

3. Are there some types of health care services that are justly distributed on the basis of the ability to pay? Should, for example, transplantable organs ever be distributed on the basis of ability to pay? It is likely that we will see the development of a totally implantable artificial heart (TIAH) within 10 years. We may potentially need 350,000 such devices annually at a cost of $150,000 each (in 1998 dollars). Because more than 70 percent of these would go to individuals over age 65, the potential cost to the Medicare program would be $35 billion a year. If it were not a Medicare-covered benefit, only the wealthy elderly would be able to afford it. Would it be unjust to deny TIAHs to Medicaid beneficiaries or the uninsured in our society or to allow individual employers to determine whether or not it would be a covered benefit in their health plans? (We owe this example to Leonard Fleck, of Michigan State University.)

HEALTH CARE REFORM

1992 Reform Efforts

In 1992, President William Clinton vowed to pursue sweeping reforms to America's health care system. Yet, in 1996, Republican candidate for president Robert Dole ridiculed Clinton's efforts as a perfect example of the bankrupt policies of big government, claiming that Clinton's plan, which never reached a congressional vote, would have "come between you and your doctor" with "hundreds of new bureaucracies" and "billions of dollars in tax increases." However, no alternative reform efforts have been accomplished in the interim except continuing efforts to reduce Medicare/Medicaid costs and a bipartisan bill sponsored by Senators Kennedy and Kassebaum designed to assure that people can keep their current insurance if they lose their jobs and to prevent insurance companies from refusing to insure people with certain preexisting medical conditions. Nothing has been done to assure that health insurance companies won't simply pass on the cost increases incurred through these limitations in excluding expensive risk-bearing customers. For this and other reasons it is likely that insurance costs will continue to rise. Moreover, at least for the present, increasing access to health care for the uninsured—let alone universal coverage—is not considered politically possible. So it is likely that access to health care for the uninsured will continue to be a problem well into the future.

In effect, the public debate on health care reform, which was front-page news for several years in the early 1990s, has been reduced to a fight over Medicare and Medicaid funding, with the other important issues being ignored for the most part or shifted to the states. A growing segment of the public apparently thinks that health care does not need reform. But facts suggest otherwise. It remains true that about 40 million Americans lack health insurance and therefore lack reasonable access to the health care system. It is also true that the very poor and the elderly currently have some access through Medicare and Medicaid; but many important services, such as long-term custodial care, are not covered. Current cost-containment efforts on the federal level may have the effect of transferring problems to the states. But states have limited budgets. The results of negotiations on this issue are not yet known. Access may be considerably reduced for the very poor and the elderly depending on the state one lives in. Even so, from the perspectives of care providers and institutions, the level of reimbursement for Medicare and Medicaid patients already does not usually cover the costs of treating them. So even though health care costs flood the federal budget with red ink, other patients in effect subsidize Medicare and Medicaid patients by paying higher costs.

Those costs are staggering. The United States is nearly alone among developed nations in not offering universal coverage at some level, at least to its citizens (South Africa also does not provide some form of universal coverage). Yet the United States spends more money on health care per capita than any other nation in the world. And the result is extremely mixed. While we lead the world in high-tech medicine, we have the worst record of any developed nation in infant mortality. We continue to overproduce highly trained specialists, even as we fail to meet significant shortages in family practice. Many of those who object to health care reform say they do not want bureaucracies making allocation decisions. But under current circumstances, allocation decisions are made by market forces that reward the wealthy and well-insured at the expense of everyone else. And it is difficult to argue that this approach has any plausible ethical basis.

Considerations of fairness and justice seem to require that people generally ought to have access to similar levels of health care services. Such access cannot be unlimited because needs will always outstrip resources. At the same time, it seems clear that Americans do not wish to dismantle our health care system in any fundamental way. Further, it does not seem reasonable to prohibit those who can afford it from spending their own resources on at least some very costly, risky, or marginal-benefit services that cannot be provided to all. So, at least for now, health reform amounts to the question "How can we cost-effectively provide at least an adequate level of health care services to virtually everyone who needs them?"

As we begin to explore proposals, it may be useful to keep several additional facts in mind. Six out of ten workers receive some health care benefits through their employers. Levels of coverage vary greatly, with workers in the public sector (federal, state, and local government employees) generally having better health care benefits than those in the private sector, and those in the manufacturing portion of the private sector generally having more generous benefits than employees in the service sector (the service sector is the fastest growing portion of the economy). Sixteen percent of part-time workers received benefits in 1993, while only 10 percent of businesses extend benefits to temporary employees. Approximately 73 percent of the self-employed have coverage, but most of these depend on benefits from spouses employed elsewhere. Apart from Medicare and Medicaid and their state variants, health care coverage normally comes from employer benefit plans or individual insurance policies. So the greatest portion of those currently without insurance are those employed in jobs without insurance benefits who cannot or will not afford private insurance.

The "Clinton Plan"

In 1993–94, under the general leadership of Hillary Rodham Clinton, a working group of health policy experts developed the outlines of a health care reform proposal that was intended to address the needs of the uninsured. The plan was to guarantee health coverage for all Americans by 1998 and would have included at least these benefits: coverage for routine doctor visits, hospitalization and emergency services, most preventive care, prescription drugs, rehabilitative services, home health and extended nursing care, and lab and diagnostic services. Some coverage of mental health and substance abuse services was also proposed, but not completely defined. The proposal was explicitly tied to a number of principles that were considered to express both the Clinton administration's values and minimum criteria for any alternative; the plan was to assure universal coverage, fairness, choice, responsibility, simplicity, quality, and privacy.

The plan would have required all employers to provide at least the minimum benefit package defined above, though employers had the option to offer more elaborate benefits if they chose to do so. To help small employers, the self-employed, and others to negotiate insurance rates as low as those offered large employers and groups, the Clinton plan required that states set up "health alliances" that would bargain with private insurance providers and offer other administrative services. Employers would have been required to pay at least 80 percent of the cost of the average health insurance plan for unmarried workers and 55 percent of a plan for those with families, but companies with fewer than 5,000 employers would not be obligated to contribute more than 7.9 percent of payroll. Subsidies would have been available to small companies for whom even these costs would have been a hardship. Total government contributions would have been capped and increases in the price of insurance premiums would have been held to the rate of inflation as ways of controlling costs. Further savings and efficiencies were to have been realized by issuing medical ID cards, simplifying paperwork, and increasing standardization. Policies would have been continued during lapses in employment and could not have been canceled. The program was to have been funded through a tax increase on cigarettes, a 1 percent payroll tax on large companies that did not join an alliance, and an assessment of 2.5 percent on the members of alliances.

The Clinton plan aroused heated opposition among many groups, particularly the American Medical Association and members of the health insurance industry. Even though the preservation of choice was a guiding principle among the Clinton plan's developers, widespread criticism centered on the possibility that many people would be forced to accept care providers and programs against their will by cost-conscious health alliance administrators. The alliances themselves were seen as unwarranted government (bureaucratic) interference in the affairs of private citizens, as well as an unacceptable intrusion into free enterprise. Smaller private insurers feared that they would not be able to compete for business on the level of the groups formed by alliances, while large insurers argued that vesting choices in the hands of the alliance administrators would prove anticompetitive and perhaps drive "losers" out of business. Businesses decried "employer mandates," arguing that even with limitations and subsidies, the required benefits would bankrupt many firms. And the Government Accounting Office pointed out that the plan's proposed funding sources were woefully inadequate, at the same time that Medicare and Medicaid were already on the verge of bankruptcy. Many in Congress argued that it would be foolhardy to attempt so expensive a new program when existing obligations to seniors and the needy already could not be met.

In retrospect, it seems clear that some of these criticisms were more apt than others. Certainly it is true that the advocates of the Clinton plan never made clear how it was to be funded without a politically unacceptable tax increase of great proportions. However, questions about how much the plan would have limited patients' choices and about the extent and propriety of government intrusion and bureaucracy are much harder to assess because they are really matters of differing social and political philosophy. After all, many people who have benefits under the current system are being "forced" by economic or other considerations into HMOs or other care-delivery systems that they would not have chosen for themselves. And the examples of Medicare and Medicaid provide ammunition for arguments both for and against the involvement of the federal government in health care. Some critics saw in the Clinton plan the first steps toward socialized medicine. It can also be argued that the Clinton plan was torpedoed in large measure by those in the insurance industry whom the plan's developers were trying hard to protect. After all, other reformers who advocated a single-payer system, something potentially much closer to socialized medicine, because of its greater cost effectiveness really would have put most private insurers out of business. In any event, with the failure of this and other plans for health care reform, the Clinton administration publicly backed away from any but incremental efforts toward its original ambitious goals.

Republican Leadership Proposals

Until the Clinton plan was swamped by budget problems and negative publicity, health care reform continued to be an issue with a seemingly vast constituency. Accordingly, other government leaders, including many Republicans, offered alternative approaches to the problems of health care. These proposals differed in many details, but shared a number of common themes. First, these plans shared an opposition to employer mandates, preferring incentives, voluntary purchasing alliances, and other unspecified noncoercive measures to encourage companies to offer benefits to their employees. Second, even more than the advocates of the Clinton plan, the House and Senate leadership strongly opposed tax hikes to support or subsidize coverage, except for increased taxes on cigarettes (those who play also pay). Instead, it was widely argued that cuts in Medicare and Medicaid, and other efficiencies, would prove sufficient to provide funding for health care reform. Third, these plans shared an emphasis on choice of providers and private insurers and a distaste for federal regulation or oversight. However, fourth, most were willing to require that coverage not be denied people because of preexisting conditions and that it not be lost during transitions between jobs or short-term family emergencies.

Critics of these proposals objected that voluntary measures were unlikely to accomplish much for the 40 million Americans without health care coverage because employers continued to insist that costs for even minimal insurance coverage were far out of reach, particularly in the case of small-business owners. Thus, unless the government was prepared to subsidize such coverage heavily, something philosophically and economically unwelcome to the House and Senate leadership, only a few businesses with well-developed social consciences could be expected to sign on. Second, it has proved impossible to cut Medicare and Medicaid enough to extract savings that could be put to other health care needs. As passage of the Kennedy-Kassebaum bill proved, there was consensus on portability of coverage and on protecting people from uninsurability due to certain preexisting conditions. However, the leadership proposals did little or nothing to restrain the growth in health care costs. On the contrary, critics contended, preventing insurers from excluding high-risk clients from coverage could only drive up costs for the rest of the population.

In the end, none of the incentives or other measures intended to get employers to provide benefits voluntarily have been enacted. Instead, as the magnitude of the Medicare/Medicaid crisis loomed larger, along with the welfare reform issue with which Medicaid was sometimes associated, attention turned elsewhere. And, as predicted, there has been no rush on the part of employers to provide expanded benefits to their employees. Instead, even during a period of unprecedented economic growth, efforts continue to roll back benefit levels in many sectors of the business community.

Rationing

The goals of health care reform involve both increasing access and restraining costs. As the national effort to reform health care loses political support, it seems increasingly likely that most of the battles over this issue will occur at the state level. Some states have already taken innovative steps to address health care reform. One approach, the Oregon Plan, involves rationing, in combination with employer requirements to cover every employee working more than 17.5 hours per week. The basic principle of the Oregon Health Plan is to rank-order the most important and cost-effective health care services and then offer as many of them as the budget will allow to every uninsured citizen. Whatever services cannot be paid for by the state are the responsibility of those who want and can afford them. But at least those formerly without any financial access to the health care system, originally some 120,000 people, are assured a decent minimum of services.

The Oregon Health Plan (the Plan) covers U.S. citizens and legal aliens who are Oregon residents, with incomes less than 100 percent of the federal poverty level, or 133 percent for pregnant women and children under age 6. What services are covered was originally determined by a public and legislative process that rank-ordered more than 700 diagnosis/treatment pairs according to utilitarian considerations of extent, quality, and duration of benefit; the number of people affected; cost-effectiveness; and public opinion. Initially, 563 of these diagnosis/treatment pairs were funded. In a 1995 revision, more diagnosis/treatment pairs were added to the list, and 606 were funded. However, increasing budget pressures and resistance to additional taxation are currently pushing the Plan into deficits and reductions in covered services.

The Plan offered services in four main areas, corresponding to four headings of Medicaid funding. In Reproductive Services, family planning, counseling, pre- and postnatal care, labor and delivery services, and home care were all covered, while infertility counseling and in vitro fertilization were not. Health Promotion and Disease Prevention was given a high priority. Immunizations, screening, and nutritional supplements ranked highest, with Pap smears, mammograms, and education about sexually transmissible diseases, smoking and drug abuse, safety, and eating disorders also supported. In the area of Chronic Disease Management, procedures or therapies that can restore full or near complete restoration of function or independence ranked highest, followed by maintaining patients in the least restrictive, most appropriate environment, including therapy, home, and respite care. But procedures regarded as futile, especially in circumstances at the end of life, were not given a high priority. Finally, in the area of Acute Illness and Episodic Treatment, diagnosis and treatment, trauma and emergency care, anesthesia and appropriate surgeries, preventive and restorative dental care, and rehabilitation for improvement of function were all covered. Therapy for alcohol and drug abuse, foot care for the elderly, routine eye and hearing care, routine dental care for adults, and organ transplantations were ranked much lower and in many cases were not covered.

The ethical basis of the Oregon Health Plan combines some considerations of fairness with an explicitly utilitarian rationale. Generally, children and programs related to children were favored over programs directed toward the elderly because the duration of benefits is much greater, cost is often lower, and the probability of benefit is higher (many elderly patients respond to treatment less successfully than most children). Programs that benefit many people were favored over programs that address concerns of a small number of people, even if the minority considered the issue to be important. And health problems that seem attributable to unwise personal choices or irresponsibility tended to be less favorably ranked. Advocates of the Oregon approach consider that, especially since public funds are concerned, these priorities, which express widely held public health policy beliefs, are much as they should be. Critics, however, objected to the Plan on many grounds.

QUESTIONS FOR DISCUSSION

1. During the debates leading to the Democratic primary elections between Vice President Gore and former Senator Bradley in 1999–2000, each offered plans designed to address some aspects of the American health care crisis. What plans did each offer? What were the advantages and disadvantages of each proposal? Are any initiatives currently under consideration? What are they?

2. *Case 7.5: When Does Care Become Futile?*—Elizabeth is a 73-year-old woman who has expressive aphasia and left-sided dysfunction as a result of strokes she experienced when she was 62. She lives with her daughter and son-in-law, who care for her. She is confined to bed and/or a wheelchair, but is able to feed herself.

   Elizabeth has just been admitted to the coronary care unit following an acute heart attack. She undergoes a thorough examination, and the cardiologist determines that she might benefit from a bypass operation. Elizabeth's daughter is asked to approve the operation. Bearing in mind that one reason for the high cost of care in the United States is performance of procedures some might regard as unnecessary, are there any ethical issues involved in this situation? What would you decide if you were Elizabeth's daughter? Would your answer be affected if Elizabeth had acute dementia? If Elizabeth had end-stage liver disease? If Elizabeth were entirely uninsured? Discuss.

3. As mentioned in the text, the United States is virtually the only economically developed nation not to offer its citizens near universal access to health care at some level. Why do you think this is? Research the health care system of one or more of the other industrialized nations, such as the United Kingdom, Canada, Germany, or Japan. Do any of those systems suggest directions the United States ought to take?

CHAPTER EIGHT

The Ethics of Euthanasia and Assisted Suicide

PHYSICIAN-ASSISTED SUICIDE

On June 4, 1990, Dr. Jack Kevorkian, a retired pathologist from Michigan, provided Alzheimer's disease sufferer Janet Adkins (at her request) with a simple way to administer a lethal poison to herself. Their actions aroused a considerable uproar in medical and legal communities, as well as among those interest groups with a stake in "right-to-life" or "right-to-die" issues. Years later, this controversy has not ended.

> *In April 1999, Jack Kevorkian was convicted and imprisoned for second-degree murder and delivery of a controlled substance for the death of Thomas Youk. When Kevorkian directly injected Thomas Youk with a lethal substance, Kevorkian moved beyond physician-assisted suicide, as the term is usually used, and performed active euthanasia. This death was videotaped and played over national television. Kevorkian's actions have made thoughtful and less sensational discussions of end-of-life issues harder to hear.*

Almost all professional organizations in the health care field, right-to-life advocates, the Roman Catholic Church, and many others adamantly opposed Dr. Kevorkian's actions and assisted suicide in general. The actual number of his public supporters is small. Yet polls show that majorities of people are in favor of at least some forms of assisted suicide; and at least one state, Oregon, has passed legislation permitting physicians to assist some of their patients to die. When the issue of help in dying is separated from the personality and actions of Dr. Kevorkian, a very large number of health care providers share a deep sense that some form of assistance in dying might be justifiable when terminal patients are suffering uncontrollably or have subsided into vegetative states.

135

In this chapter, we explore ethical questions about euthanasia, and we examine some of Dr. Kevorkian's actions. After preliminary discussion, we outline several cases to help focus our thinking. While some of these cases are related to those of people Dr. Kevorkian has assisted to die, no assumptions should be made about whether they accurately portray the individuals involved. Simply, the details of their medical histories are not public knowledge. We are attempting to think about ethical issues from the perspective of participating in public policy decisions rather than praising or blaming Jack Kevorkian. Because of his high profile in connection with this issue, we conclude with a brief discussion of ethical concerns about Dr. Kevorkian's activities in assisting suicides.

EUTHANASIA

Types of Euthanasia

Let's start by defining some standard terminology to help identify ethically relevant differences among euthanasia cases. The Greek roots of the term *euthanasia* mean a "good death," but beyond this meaning, the word is used in various ways. *Active euthanasia* means killing or actively taking steps to cause death. *Passive euthanasia* means not doing something that would slow or stop a patient's dying, thereby allowing the patient to die. Some writers further distinguish between withholding (not starting) treatment, which they consider passive euthanasia, versus withdrawing (stopping) a treatment that is already underway, which they consider active euthanasia. A legal and ethical consensus has developed that competent patients and some other decision makers, such as close family members, do have the right to refuse and discontinue treatment, even when doing so will lead to death. So this distinction has come to seem less important than it once did.

> *The primary accrediting agency for health care organizations (JCAHO) has written standards of care that address end-of-life issues. Advance directives are documents that delineate people's individual preferences for medical interventions should they become unable to participate in care decisions. Advance directives guide medical decision making but cannot be legally enforced in most states. So-called living wills can specify patients' wishes concerning a much broader spectrum of issues, including who is to make decisions concerning their care. Living wills are legally binding in only a few states.*

We also distinguish between *voluntary euthanasia*, which involves a competent patient's giving his or her informed consent, and *nonvoluntary euthanasia*, when the patient is not competent to provide consent for him- or herself, perhaps because the patient is in a coma. *Involuntary euthanasia* would be a case in which a competent patient does not ask for euthanasia but is, nevertheless, killed. This is simply murder, and no morally responsible person has ever argued for anything like it. Finally, *assisted euthanasia* means that someone other than the patient is actively or passively involved in the causal chain leading to the patient's death. *Physician-assisted suicide,* as the term has come to be used in the aftermath of Jack Kevorkian's activities, is one form of assisted euthanasia in which a physician provides a simple means for a person to commit suicide under the supervision of that physician.

These standard definitions can lead to some uncomfortable consequences, especially for those who consider all euthanasia to be ethically unacceptable. For example, according to these definitions, a patient who competently refuses a life-sustaining treatment is engaged in euthanasia (voluntary passive). So is a physician who, with the full approval of a patient's family, elects not to attempt yet another effort to resuscitate an unconscious dying patient (nonvoluntary passive). Similarly, a physician who, with the consent of the family, elects not to initiate another course of chemotherapy because it seems futile in an incompetent terminal patient is also engaging in nonvoluntary passive euthanasia. A patient who intentionally removes the feeding tube that is keeping him alive because he has "had enough" and then refuses to permit it to be reinserted is committing voluntary active euthanasia. Few opponents of euthanasia would be likely to argue against these actions in these circumstances; probably most people, including those who are uncomfortable with some forms of euthanasia, would not judge these examples to be ethically wrong. Indeed, few people actually oppose *all* forms of euthanasia. To most people, particularly when extraordinary measures are being taken to prolong an imminently terminal, painful, or unconscious death, these kinds of euthanasia do not seem morally abhorrent.

Dying is a normal life process. All living things die because they are alive. Are there ethical issues that should be recognized when the dying process is stopped?

We need to ask whether there are good ethical grounds to oppose all forms of euthanasia. People who hold this position sometimes say "We have no right to play God with another human life," or "All life is sacred." Critics of this position respond that we are already playing God. We play God just as much by artificially prolonging a painful or unconscious death as we would do by stopping our interference or changing its nature.

Moreover, even euthanasia's most outspoken opponents do not really mean that all life is sacred. At most, these outspoken opponents mean that all human life is sacred and perhaps only innocent human life is undeserving of death. When we go on to ask what makes human life sacred, the answer is likely to have reference to the unique value of a human soul or person. But the soul or person of a dying patient may no longer be present at all during the final stages of physical death, as with brain-dead patients whose hearts and lungs are still working. In that case, assisting a patient's body to die would not seem wrong because the person (*soul*) is already dead.

Defining death has become problematic as technology has advanced. Prior to our ability to monitor the activity of the brain, cessation of breathing and heartbeat meant death. So, a person who breathed and had a heartbeat was alive even though he or she was unconscious. Then the idea of brain death developed. This meant that a person who was previously considered alive because of respiration and heart activity was now dead if his or her brain did not demonstrate appropriate activity. Current practice in many states permits either criterion to determine death: permanent cessation of either full brain function or cardiopulmonary function.

How parallel is the case of brain death to the case of a persistent vegetative state? Determining the presence of a soul is not an easy matter, but it is surely possible that it would not continue to exist in well-established, persistent vegetative states in the absence of consciousness. And, if that is the case, it would not seem obviously wrong to end the maintenance of the body through some form of euthanasia.

Obviously, this discussion does not settle the issue. The "slippery slope" argument is that if any form of euthanasia is permitted, even a limited or regulated one, it will become impossible to prevent wanton abuse of patients by means of other forms of euthanasia. Of course, this argument is a little dangerous, because it implies that some forms of euthanasia may be moral. It would be the other cases, the wantonly abusive cases that such permissiveness might lead to, that would be ethically wrong. But we cannot simply dismiss this concern. Surely the potential for abuse of euthanasia by exhausted, despairing, or merely greedy relatives cannot be ignored.

What Makes Euthanasia Ethically Troubling?

Euthanasia is ethically troubling because it unavoidably involves conflicting values. As health care professionals, we want to preserve life, yet we also want to respect the wishes of patients and families to control their own end-of-life decisions, even if they choose to end their lives. We want to stop patients from suffering, yet we also know that there are cases where nothing that is acceptable to the patient short of death will stop suffering. We want to do everything possible for our patients, yet we also know that "doing everything" can be futile, a matter of simply prolonging a death. We want to protect our patients from undue pressure to die prematurely, yet we want to permit patients and families wide latitude to decide on how their end-of-life care will be managed.

Most foes of euthanasia oppose active, rather than passive, euthanasia because it involves killing, and so it seems close to murder. Much law has been framed along these lines, with active euthanasia generally being thought of as murder, and passive being regarded as not criminal. Unfortunately, there is no clear guidance on how to draw this line between active and passive, either in the law or elsewhere. Patients already have the right to refuse or discontinue treatment, even when doing so will lead to their deaths; but actively discontinuing treatment can be active euthanasia. And there are many other examples that blur this line between active and passive. Does failing to replenish the supply of a feeding tube constitute an active intervention or a passive withholding of life support? Would failing to restart an intravenous pump or respirator during a power outage count as active or passive? Many health professionals can see no relevant difference and no ethically important distinction between active and passive euthanasia in cases like these—or in general. When artificial means are all that keeps the patient going, letting the patient die almost always involves actively doing something. Therefore, many health professionals who can accept passive euthanasia also accept active euthanasia under some circumstances, because there just does not seem to be much difference.

Some critics of euthanasia think the most important issue is intent to kill: ethically wrong, active euthanasia would be actions taken with the intent to kill the patient, whereas ethically acceptable, passive euthanasia would be a by-product of responsible actions such as pain relief or hydration. (Hydration and pain control can have the effect of hastening death.) But can distinctions between ethically acceptable and unacceptable actions at the end of life be drawn according to such changeable and elusive things as intentions? Aren't end-of-life motivations often deeply mixed? When I want Mr. A.'s suffering to end, and I know that giving him a certain level of pain medication is not only likely to reduce his suffering but also to hasten his death, don't I also, in effect at least, intend his death?

However, and in some ways this is the really operative point, passive euthanasia—withholding of extraordinary therapies—does not always yield results that are in the patient's best interests. Is it really morally better to allow a terminal patient with uncontrolled pain to suffer while untreated, but treatable, infections finally kill him (that is, "passively let him die") than to err on the side of early, painless intervention? There are myriad ways to hasten death and make it less painful. There are diseases, nervous inflammations, dementias so horrible that they offer no remotely plausible hint of meaningful life, but only unrelieved and lengthy suffering. Is it obvious that even relatively ordinary measures ought to be undertaken to preserve such horrors? One of the most deeply rooted principles of health care is to seek always to act so as to produce the most merciful (beneficial) outcome under the circumstances. In circumstances like these, active euthanasia can seem ethically justifiable.

It is sometimes tempting to say that if "extraordinary measures" are withdrawn, then we don't have euthanasia. However, as the limits of life-sustaining, transplantation, and other forms of technology develop and become more widely used, it becomes harder and harder to know what counts as "extraordinary measures." Traditional definitions of extraordinary measures provide little guidance in many cases, because they rely on vague terms such as what is "burdensome" or "excessive." Many also presuppose that patients are competent to make judgements about what is and what is not excessive or burdensome, when in fact many such patients are in no position to do this. But if we cannot find a clear sense of what an extraordinary measure is, how can the "no extraordinary measures" criterion be applied?

The idea of what is appropriate treatment continues to evolve as new medications, therapies, and technologies are developed. For example, surgical intervention in utero was not possible in the 1960s but is possible now. The point is that what constitutes extraordinary measures is dynamic and ever-changing.

References to other medical codes of ethics, including the Hippocratic oath, do little to provide guidance. The oath does prohibit giving or suggesting deadly drugs. But a large majority of the drugs routinely prescribed by physicians can be deadly; that is one reason their distribution is restricted. Moreover, quite ordinary measures, such as providing hydration or controlling pain, can hasten death—would Hippocrates really want to promote dehydration or prohibit pain control? Besides, as we have already seen, the Hippocratic oath is widely viewed as expressing values rather than defining acceptable practice. After all, it also prohibits physicians from performing surgery ("using the knife").

To some, the most important distinction is not between active and passive euthanasia or between ordinary versus extraordinary means. The most important distinction is between voluntary and other forms of euthanasia, because what is crucial is the patient's consent. It is obvious that involuntary euthanasia, euthanizing a competent person without his or her consent, is simply murder.

> *One American value is that of self-determination. Advance directives are an attempt to extend self-determination to those times when the person is unable to speak for himself or herself. But what about persons who have not attained legal age? Or those individuals who are no longer considered to be legally competent to exercise self-determination?*

So perhaps the competence of the patient making the request is crucial. Indeed, practice in the Netherlands, where active, voluntary euthanasia, though not legal, is not prosecuted, and legislation in Oregon both restrict euthanasia to circumstances in which a competent (in Oregon, terminal) patient makes repeated, documented requests for assistance in dying. Similarly, the Second and Ninth Circuit Courts (New York and Washington, respectively) have handed down decisions that in effect permitted physicians to prescribe life-ending medications for use by terminally ill, competent patients who wished to hasten their own deaths. The Second Circuit's decision was based primarily on the idea of equal protection: statutes prohibiting persons in the final stages of terminal illness from assistance in ending life lack any rational basis when at the same time comparable patients are allowed to hasten their deaths by forgoing life-support systems. The Ninth Circuit's decision was based on "liberty interests." That court found that "Matters involving the most intimate and personal choices a person may make in a lifetime, choices central to personal dignity and autonomy, are central to the liberty protected by the fourteenth amendment." Such choices, the court found, may include voluntary euthanasia.

However, on June 26th, 1997, the U.S. Supreme Court dealt a blow to the hopes of "death with dignity" advocates by finding against the circuit courts in each case. In *Washington et al. v. Harold Glucksberg*, the Court pointed out that while "attitudes toward suicide itself have changed . . . our laws have consistently condemned and continue to prohibit, assisting suicide. Despite changes in medical technology and notwithstanding an increased emphasis on the importance of end of life decision making, we have not retreated from this prohibition." While reasserting "the right of a competent individual to refuse medical treatment," the Court cited a number of other arguments against legalizing physician-assisted suicide, including the likelihood that a decision to end one's life would often be driven by psychiatric illness, such as severe depression associated with uncontrolled pain. Thus, the choice to commit suicide to eliminate unbearable pain would not necessarily be a *competent* one.

Our purpose in this chapter is to discuss the ethics of euthanasia and physician-assisted suicide rather than its legal basis. Moreover, legal or not, euthanasia, both as an issue or as a practice, will not disappear. Nevertheless, the Supreme Court is quite right that assessment of competence in end-of-life cases can be extremely difficult. Terminal patients *are* often profoundly depressed, and their depression can undermine any sense of value that continued living might otherwise offer. Moreover, terminal or not, when pain management is inadequate, patients can hardly focus on anything else. They may prefer death to continued suffering, even if there is some likelihood that their suffering will eventually be controlled or even that they will recover. However, when pain control is adequate, this chemical intervention can seriously interfere with patients' abilities to judge their own prospects and circumstances. The importance of respecting patient autonomy looms significantly when voluntary euthanasia is under consideration, but determining when autonomy is sufficiently impaired that honoring a patient's choice may not be in that patient's best interests is problematic.

Morally relevant, convincing distinctions among various kinds of euthanasia can be difficult to draw, yet many people are far more willing to regard some cases of euthanasia as ethically acceptable than others. Certainly the fear that euthanasia can be abused is an important consideration, and the responsibilities involved in making life-and-death decisions are always morally stringent. But in cases in which meaningful life is impossible, in which death is imminent, in which unendurable pain cannot be adequately controlled, many people seem to believe that a merciful death is to be hoped for and, perhaps, brought about.

CASES OF PHYSICIAN-ASSISTED SUICIDE

Abstract discussion is rarely sufficient to clarify issues. Perhaps it will now be more useful to look at some specific cases. These cases resemble those of actual patients who contacted Jack Kevorkian and asked him to assist them to die. However, there is a great deal about the real-life cases of those patients that cannot be known and that would be relevant to a full understanding of the ethical issues involved. Accordingly, it is crucial to remember that the goal of this section is to clarify our thinking about euthanasia rather than to condemn or commend Jack Kevorkian.

Case 8.1: Patient with Mild Dementia

Janet A., 54, is suffering from Alzheimer's disease, a progressive generalized deterioration of the brain, accompanied by diminished capacities for memory, judgment, thought, and self-determination. Janet is seriously distressed by her increasing dependence on others and her rapidly eroding abilities to engage in meaningful activities. She lacks the financial resources to situate herself in an assisted-care facility, and does not wish to do so anyway. Instead, she is seeking physician-assisted suicide.

Case 8.2: Patient with Chronic Disease and Pain

Judith C., a 42-year-old wife and mother of two, has a long history of psychiatric problems, including severe depression and anxiety. Over a period of years, she has been addicted to painkillers and anti-anxiety drugs and has become obese (to the point that she is confined to a wheelchair and largely unable to care for herself). She is also diagnosed with chronic fatigue syndrome and fibromyalgia, a painful disease related to the immune system. She is still taking medications for these conditions. In spite of her husband's opposition, Judith, too, is seeking physician-assisted suicide.

Case 8.3: Patient with Terminal Illness and Pain

Marcella L., 67, is suffering unrelenting pain from end-stage emphysema and congestive heart disease, a condition regarded as terminal (that is, likely to end in death within six months and probably sooner). All forms of pain management short of induced unconsciousness appear insufficient to relieve her suffering, and Marcella drifts in and out of a coma-like stupor only to cry and whimper in constant pain. She has long since registered her request not to be resuscitated in the event of heart failure, a desire with which her family fully concurs.

Case 8.4: Patient in Persistent Vegetative State

Rodney M., 84, has lapsed into a persistent vegetative state due to a stroke, the most recent of several he has experienced in the past few years. Because he had not registered any preferences concerning his end-of-life care and has no known relatives, he is still being given assistance in respiration, as well as nutrition through a naso-gastric tube. His condition has been progressive without being life-threatening. His physician believes that he will be stable indefinitely, provided that his care is continued.

There are many differences among these four cases. While some people may think that none of these patients would be good candidates for any form of assistance in dying, others may think that least some of them deserve what is sometimes called "death with dignity." People who believe that any assistance in dying is unethical would hold that assisting these individuals to die would be morally wrong; however, most people would feel quite uncomfortable about lumping all four patients into a single category. And, in fact, all four of these patients, as well as others like them, have been euthanized.

Janet A.'s suicide (case 8.1) would probably have been an instance of active, voluntary, assisted euthanasia. In her case, so far as we know, Dr. Kevorkian did not actually administer the fatal injection, though he installed the intravenous line by which it was made; he only encouraged and enabled Adkins to do so. Still, for our purposes, we may agree to count this as a case of (physician-) assisted voluntary euthanasia. What can be said about the morality of such actions?

The American Medical Association rejects active euthanasia, whether voluntary or involuntary. Accordingly, the AMA rejects Kevorkian's actions as unprofessional and unethical practice and would counsel against Janet A.'s request. The AMA endorses and actually restricts use of the term *euthanasia* to passive deaths of patients who are terminally ill, especially when they are in pain or in persistent vegetative states and when *extraordinary measures* are involved in sustaining life. But, remember, there is no universally accepted understanding of the term extraordinary measures. So the clearest case of euthanasia the AMA could accept would be one in which a physician, with the informed consent of all parties with legal standing, refrains from undertaking an extraordinary measure to lengthen the dying of a terminally ill patient who is persistently vegetative or suffering. As we will see, none of our cases quite fits this description.

Those who are willing to regard Janet A.'s physician-assisted suicide as ethically acceptable are most likely to reason from a perspective that emphasizes the value of individual autonomy. Although Janet A. was developing Alzheimer's disease, her case was, we may assume, not so far advanced that she would have been incapable of fully informed consent. (In fact, she left a handwritten letter explaining her decision, something that many advocates of a right to die find compelling evidence of her soundness of mind.) Unless there are other valid reasons to override her wishes, then, some might argue that it was not clearly wrong to respect Janet A.'s wishes in this matter.

On the other hand, Janet A. was not suffering from a terminal illness, nor was she actually in uncontrollable pain. In fact, she was not yet a burden to others, though she feared she would become one. So what exactly was the problem that led Janet to request assistance in dying? To all appearances, it was fear, together with increasing difficulties in living.

Under normal circumstances, what Janet A. might have needed most was not assistance in dying, but sympathetic counseling, supportive home care, and, perhaps, spiritual support and human companionship.

Janet A. might not have found her life worth living even with all this in place. But it is not obvious, even if she remained convinced that her own suicide was her best option, that others had any ethical justification for helping her commit suicide. Even if Janet herself had a moral right to kill herself, others may not have had a moral responsibility or even a moral justification to assist her. Unless others had good reason to think she had exhausted all reasonable options and was not acting out of depression, they might have had an ethical obligation, not only not to help, but also to try to prevent Janet A. from committing suicide.

From a virtue ethics perspective, it is difficult to justify or condemn Janet's choice. Though advocates might paint her desire not to be burdensome to others and to face her own death as thoughtful and courageous, it can also look self-centered and cowardly. There is also the precedent her actions set, which, depending on one's point of view can be positive, in giving people control over their own deaths, or negative, in encouraging people who fear deterioration and being burdensome to others to kill themselves.

It is important to emphasize again that those who support some sort of death with dignity or a patient's freedom to choose do not have to regard Janet A.'s decision or Jack Kevorkian's involvement as ethically justifiable. We might also agree that their actions had the effect of placing assistance-in-dying issues before the public without agreeing that their actions in themselves were ethically appropriate. So, thinking specifically about the case of Janet A., and leaving aside many other issues tangential to that case, the most likely line of argument for those who wish to find it ethically acceptable would emphasize the importance of individual autonomy. Those opposed would probably argue that many other good alternatives had not been adequately explored, perhaps because of a desire to use this patient for political purposes.

Judith C.'s case (8.2) presents some new questions. First, chronic fatigue syndrome is not fatal, though it is frustrating (a friend who has it describes her experience as a case of the flu that has gone on for two and a half years). Fibromyalgia involves muscle and connective tissue pain, which "occurs mainly in females, may be induced or intensified by physical or mental stress, poor sleep, trauma, exposure to dampness or cold, and occasionally by a systemic, usually rheumatic, disorder" (*Merck Manual*, 1992, p. 1370). At least under most circumstances, the actual pain of fibromyalgia can be adequately controlled by "reassurance and explanation of the benign nature of the syndrome, as well as stretching exercises, improved sleep, local applications of heat, gentle massage, and low-dose tricyclic agents at bedtime . . . to promote deeper sleep" (*Merck Manual*, 1992, p. 1370). Neither chronic fatigue syndrome nor fibromyalgia present the prospect of progressive deterioration or hopelessness for recovery or improvement that typical Alzheimer's cases do. So there is at least some reason to think that Judith C.'s medical problems were less intractable than those of many other patients who might consider assistance in dying.

Second, her history of psychiatric problems, her depression and anxiety, and her (past) addiction to painkilling and anti-anxiety drugs all raise serious doubts about her ability to make fully competent decisions, especially life-threatening ones. Her physical disabilities might well have compounded her sense of despair, giving her an unreasonably gloomy assessment of her circumstances. Judith's husband publicly opposed her desire for assistance in dying. And, while Judith herself might have been deeply depressed and felt her life was not worth living, her husband and her two children probably did not share that view.

Given her long history of psychological problems, it is not unreasonable to suppose that the etiology of Judith's muscle pain might have been psychogenic, though that would not render it unreal. Without more information, it is also difficult to know what to make of her dependence on pain- and anxiety-controlling drugs. It might be that the pain Judith experienced was greater than what could be managed by the normal, innocuous therapies of heat, massage, and aspirin. But it is also possible that Judith exaggerated her pain because she found the medications numbed her depression. Without more information, such judgments can only be speculation.

Nevertheless, it would be hard to argue that Judith was a good candidate for assistance in dying. She was clearly capable of meaningful life, and her prognosis was neither terminal nor degenerative, nor even, by many measures, terribly bad. Whatever Judith herself may have thought, the actual suffering which she experienced did not seem to be of an order of magnitude comparable to the worst sorts of pain undergone by some cancer patients, for example, or sufferers from kidney stones. She was clearly depressed and may have been impaired in her decision-making capacities by medications. And her family did not wish her to die.

Who, then, would argue that assisting Judith C. to die in these circumstances was an ethically defensible act of euthanasia? Jack Kevorkian did assist her suicide, saying, in an interview with NBC's Chris Hansen (*Dateline*, August 24, 1996), "She was incapacitated, in a wheelchair; she couldn't take care of herself . . . she was ill. Her doctor said all she could do is go into a nursing home. It [the justification for assisting in suicide] has nothing to do with lethality [or a patient's medical condition]. It's quality of life, Chris, it's quality of life!" But it is difficult to see that this situation presented a quality of life so unendurable as to justify killing Judith C., or assisting her to kill herself, in spite of her request. To suppose otherwise seems to place so much weight on the "face value" of individual autonomy that virtually nothing else is taken into consideration, while at the same time ignoring evidence that Judith C. was not necessarily competent to exercise anything like that kind of autonomy.

By contrast, Marcella L. (case 8.3) exhibited many characteristics that some advocates of limited forms of euthanasia consider sufficient to justify assistance in dying. Her condition was hopeless of improvement and terminal. She was unable to manage her pain without experiencing significant impairment, so that her condition varied only between unconsciousness and agony. She had a long-standing, presumably competent request not to be resuscitated, and her family supported this decision.

It is important to mention at this point that, even in those states with "living will" legislation (and not all have it), health care personnel are not generally compelled by law to follow the wishes expressed in such documents. What living wills normally do is provide information and legally protect health care personnel who do follow the wishes of the patient. They can, however, be overridden by family, others with legal standing, or by the best judgment of physicians and others. So Marcella's presumably autonomous request may have had moral authority, but there was no guarantee it would have been honored, even if all family agreed with her wishes. But in this situation, her expressed wishes would surely increase the weight of argument in favor of euthanasia. The rest of the argument would probably rest on autonomy and consequentialist factors.

Those who would argue against euthanasia in this case might argue that a patient's preferences prior to her terminal condition may not be an absolutely reliable guide to her present wishes and that perhaps one ought to err on the side of preservation of life. But is there any reason to think that she would have changed her stated wishes? Is there any reason why her suffering would create in her some new desire to live under these conditions? Or should we think that keeping Marcella alive would have involved some redemptive value in her suffering during her waning days, for her or for others, regardless of her desire to live? Whatever we may think, these arguments would have weakened as she subsided into incapacity for higher mental function and her personality was extinguished by suffering or medication. And we need to be careful. If suffering is redemptive and inspires a desire to live regardless of what a patient says she wants, and assuming we want to promote redemption of souls, then what is the justification for relieving suffering under any circumstances? Wouldn't relieving a patient's suffering reduce the saving effects of that suffering? Yet, it is not reasonable to be too dogmatically certain that Marcella's experiences had no value, or only a negative one.

But in case 8.4, Rodney M. had lapsed into a persistent vegetative state due to a series of strokes, so the best evidence is that he had, at the very most, only rudimentary experiences if any at all. He was not imminently terminal, assuming there is no other pathology present. Not having expressed his wishes concerning such a situation, the question of whether to continue feeding and respiratory assistance amounts to the question of whether nonvoluntary euthanasia is justifiable in the kind of case in which the situation arises most frequently. Whether withdrawing life support is active euthanasia depends on whether Rodney's death would be seen as occurring from natural causes or from withdrawal of the support.

Arguments in favor of withdrawing support cannot depend on respecting Rodney's autonomy, because Rodney was incapable of exercising autonomy in the circumstances and had not expressed his wishes previously. Rodney's central nervous system function had deteriorated beyond rudimentary consciousness and he was not suffering. So arguments allowing euthanasia cannot be based on the desire to relieve suffering.

Instead, arguments for nonvoluntary euthanasia (apart from respecting family wishes) normally rest on consequentialist issues, together, perhaps, with considerations of social justice. Futile care eats up a huge portion of the available funds for health care; estimates have run as high as 20 percent. Given a limited budget and typical reimbursement levels substantially below hospital costs, continuing Rodney's care would have impaired our ability to provide services for others whose benefits were much clearer. Indeed, some ethicists have argued that it is unjust to these others to deprive them of services because the necessary resources have been absorbed without producing comparable benefit.

Arguments against nonvoluntary euthanasia normally rest on deontological principles, such as the sanctity of life, nonabandonment, or the intrinsic wrongness of killing. As we've already noted, however, it is interesting to think seriously about what makes life sacred or what makes killing in this instance intrinsically wrong. There is also a kind of consequentialist argument that allowing euthanasia without the patient's consent creates a climate of disrespect for life that can easily slide down a slope of increasing callousness to other forms of abuse.

Like all slippery slope arguments, however, this one tends to undermine the claim that euthanasia in Rodney's case is absolutely wrong.

CONCERNING DR. KEVORKIAN

In April 1999, after nine years, five trials, and 130 acknowledged assisted suicides, Jack Kevorkian was finally imprisoned following his conviction on charges of second-degree murder and delivering a controlled substance in his active euthanasia of Thomas Youk. While Kevorkian's imprisonment may silence this most-well-known assisted-suicide advocate, some advocates of euthanasia continue to give credit to Dr. Kevorkian for forcing the issue of assisted suicide to the forefront of public debate, even considering him a kind of martyr. Yet there is much that is ethically troubling about his activities. Bearing in mind that we do not know all about those whom Dr. Kevorkian has assisted, we still suspect he cannot have had complete access to the medical records of those whom he assisted because his licenses had been suspended and he was therefore dependent on his patients, anecdotal information, and whatever cooperation he may have received from their physicians. Moreover, he outspokenly rejected any need for collaboration or review by other physicians more familiar with each case. Yet his own training and experience in practice as a pathologist offer no assurance that his diagnostic understanding is reliable, and his unwillingness to tolerate any form of review from "idiots" who might disagree with him suggests an unconscionable level of arrogance.

Because of his eagerness to call attention to his activities as a way to promote his assisted-suicide agenda, Dr. Kevorkian is no respecter of patient privacy, let alone "death with dignity." Even more worrisome is the likelihood that Dr. Kevorkian does not explore options other than suicide in a sufficiently positive or evenhanded way. That is, it is certainly possible to suspect that Dr. Kevorkian may encourage suicide in susceptible people in order to promote his political goals.

There is evidence that at least some suicides may have been involuntary. Hugh Gale apparently attempted to pull off the mask that dispensed the lethal gases that killed him. Also, the Oakland County medical examiner reports that "at least five of those who died this summer [1996] with Kevorkian's help were sleeping or unconscious when lethal drugs entered their bloodstream, making them unable to deliver fatal doses to themselves." If that is correct, those patients, at least, did not have physician-assisted suicide; they were actively euthanized, if not murdered. Kevorkian has always insisted he is motivated only by the desire to spare his victims suffering, a defense that was central to his acquittals from prosecution. But on the basis of available information, it appears that many of Kevorkian's victims were not suffering—at least not from any physical malady—or were not suffering very much. Besides, one of the methods Kevorkian has often used to euthanize patients is carbon monoxide inhalation, but carbon monoxide has no pain-relieving properties.

In only 9 of his first 40 cases were Dr. Kevorkian's patients terminal, as far as can be determined. Cases like that of Janet Adkins set a pattern. Afflicted mainly with anxiety over her progressing Alzheimer's disease, but not with actual incapacity or even serious near-term disability at the time of her suicide, Adkins—and a large majority of Kevorkian's other victims—feared eventual incapacitation and suffering, had a need for assistance in living, and suffered from depression. As Oakland County medical examiner L. J. Dragovic said, 9 of the people he evaluated who died were terminally ill, 19 were incapacitated in some way, and 3 were neither. One of those three was Marjorie Wantz, who complained of genital pain but in fact had no genital organs. In two other cases, those of Rebecca Badger and Judith Curren, the medical examiner reported there was "essentially nothing wrong with them" except a loss of hope (Lessenberry, 1996; Lowe, 1996). If that is correct, what these people needed was psychiatric help instead of assisted suicide. In any event, it does not seem ethically responsible that, as a matter of public policy, society ought to make it easier for fearful, depressed victims of progressive, degenerative illnesses to be assisted in killing themselves, particularly by someone with inadequate knowledge of their cases and a personal agenda that might well conflict with the best interests of his patients.

QUESTIONS FOR DISCUSSION

1. Are there circumstances in which you believe euthanasia is ethically justifiable? If so, what are they? If possible, outline a case with which you are personally familiar that would fit your criteria for ethically justifiable euthanasia. What, specifically, is it about these circumstances and not others that makes euthanasia ethically justifiable?

2. Opponents of euthanasia often cite fear of abuse as the basis of their concern. Are there circumstances in which you believe euthanasia can be abused? If so, what are they? If possible, outline a case with which you are personally familiar that exemplifies this kind of abuse. Is there any effective way, from a public policy standpoint, to prevent such abuse?

3. Advocates for the mentally ill point out, rightly, that some forms of mental illness are as hopeless and oppressive as some forms of physical illness, including some that have led people to request aid in dying. If you think there are some cases in which euthanasia is ethically justifiable, do you think that cases of serious mental illness might be among them? Why or why not?

4. *Case 8.5: Patient's End-of-Life Wishes*—Ernie and Ben have been close friends for years; and, since both their wives died, they have moved in together at The Woodlands, a retirement community. Both men have talked over their wishes and concerns about medical care, and if one or the other should become incapacitated, each wants the other to make decisions for his friend. Basically, both want pain management but want aggressive care only if there is a good chance for recovery. Neither has filed any legal documents regarding care because each has confidence in the other and both distrust lawyers.

   Ernie has just found Ben unconscious, with obvious difficulty breathing, on the kitchen floor. Ben is rushed to the hospital, where he is placed on life-support equipment. Next of kin, Ben's son, who has not seen his father in eight years, is called, and insists that he wants "everything done." "No, no!" pleads Ernie. "Ben never wanted any of this. He was terrified of being stuck on them damn machines. Please, please just let him go!" Assuming Ernie is entirely right about this, what should be done? What actually will be done in this situation? If Ben is kept on life support and Ernie sneaks in and "unplugs" Ben, has Ernie acted immorally? Discuss.

5. Many of those who have sought the assistance of Jack Kevorkian in dying seem to have been able to commit suicide on their own, without involving Kevorkian. Why do you think physician assistance in general, and Jack Kevorkian in particular, have become so important to people who, under other circumstances, might well have ended their own lives without the intervention of others (especially doctors)?

CHAPTER NINE

Ethical Issues in Genetic Technology

TECHNOLOGICAL ADVANCES

Since Crick and Watson's groundbreaking work on DNA, the sciences associated with genetic research have made astonishing advances. In some instances, such as in the cases of Down's syndrome and Huntington's disease, clearly identifiable anomalies in the structure of genomes (a name for the totality of genetic material of an organism) are (so far) invariably correlated with disease conditions. In other instances, such as widely publicized "markers" for some forms of breast cancer, schizophrenia, and obesity, the relationship between the genetic anomaly and subsequent condition is much less direct; symptoms will depend to a great extent on such other factors as environment and adaptive behavior. In some cases, such as Tay-Sachs disease, there is currently no cure or effective therapy: degeneration of an infant's nervous system will be lethal within three or four years. In other cases, such as PKU (phenylketonuria), the genetically based inability to metabolize an amino acid no longer has to lead to severe retardation; a special diet can enable victims to develop in a virtually normal fashion.

> Genes, *the basic units of heredity, are linear sequences of molecules forming the DNA that provides the coded instructions for expression of hereditary characteristics.*
>
> DNA *(deoxyribonucleic acid) is the primary constituent of gene-carrying chromosomes.*
>
> Genetic engineering *is a series of procedures and technologies whereby the genetic material of an organism is manipulated for the purpose of altering hereditary traits.*
>
> Genetic markers *are specific identifiable chromosomes or segments of chromosomes that can be linked to specific genetic traits or characteristics.*
> Genetic screening *employs scientific technologies to assess an individual's genetic makeup to predict defects that may be transmitted to offspring as well as susceptibility to certain diseases known to be genetically linked.*

Thus, for some, genetic technology has already meant release from a future of inevitable suffering for themselves and those they love. For many more, it means hope that understanding at least some of the genetic mechanisms of disease can lead eventually to successful therapies—cures at best or at least adjustments to foster a more or less normal life. But for many others, genetic research has provided the expectation of great suffering without any realistic hope, has led to what is, in effect, a death sentence that cannot be avoided, preceded by a long, painful deterioration. It has also led to gross invasions of privacy, agonizing decisions about whether to initiate or continue pregnancies when there is some probability that offspring will have defects, cruel discrimination in employment and health care insurance coverage, and increasingly unsympathetic social attitudes.

In this section, we explore a few of the ethical issues that have arisen through genetic research. Before current and constantly advancing understanding of genetic inheritance began to make it possible to anticipate the futures of family members and prospective offspring, people had been able to ignore responsibility for actions that resulted in the suffering of family members because they could not understand how genetic conditions were determined. With greater knowledge, however, comes greater responsibility to make genetic choices. The ethical problems we are now faced with, both as individuals and as societies, are to make those choices in ways that preserve essential ethical values and continuity of human personhood.

ISSUES IN REPRODUCTIVE AND PRENATAL TESTING

It has now become routine, when a couple is expecting a child, to offer a series of prenatal tests, such as amniocentesis (in which amniotic fluid containing fetal cells is drawn and tested, usually around the sixteenth week of gestation) and chorionic villi sampling (in which cells from the fetal part of the placenta are drawn and tested, usually after the eighth week). These tests currently provide a great deal of information about a number of problematic genetic conditions as well as many that are normally entirely benign.

> Amniocentesis *is an invasive procedure that involves the insertion of a needle through the abdominal wall of the mother, into the amniotic cavity. Approximately 20 cc (about a tablespoon) of fluid is aspirated through the needle. This fluid is then cultured for genetic and biochemical studies. Medical complications of this procedure do not occur often, but possibilities include fetal injury, hemorrhage (maternal or fetal), infection, and leaking of amniotic fluid and premature birth.*

But the entries in this genetic report card are becoming more comprehensive all the time; and, as the Human Genome Project continues, it is quite likely that tests for thousands of genetic conditions will become available. Moreover, for reasons of economy and convenience, they are likely to be bundled together. Rather than being able to pick and choose tests for specific conditions, couples will receive a broad spectrum of information, probably including information about conditions they can hardly imagine or information they may not even want. Existing tests are not entirely without risk, nor are they always accurate, and they are also not without costs. But the costs of testing are far less than the costs of providing care for newborns with serious birth defects, much less raising them for whatever duration of life their disease conditions allow. And, for those who have middle-class access to the health care system, many of these tests are already standard.

What is the implication of genetic screening and prenatal testing? Just because a technology is available, are we obligated to make use of it?

As genetic research continues, it is becoming more common to suggest that prospective parents be screened prior to conceiving children. One reason is that the largest number of genetic problems and disease conditions cannot now be cured or managed effectively. So preconception screening can help prospective parents make informed choices about the risks their genetic makeup may pose to their children. If those risks are serious enough, such partners may elect to adopt children or take other steps to avoid these problems. Other genetic conditions cannot be evaluated until after pregnancy. While testing on a developing fetus can help parents make informed choices and, if necessary, prepare for problems they may face in providing their children with the best lives possible, it can pose another set of problems.

For many prospective parents, disclosure of a serious problem will inevitably lead to consideration of abortion. While no responsible genetic counselor will normally suggest abortion (it would be too directive), there is no need to do so; in today's climate, the issue is unavoidable. It is not unusual for obstetricians to tell couples that "If you wouldn't consider aborting on the basis of what you find out, you probably shouldn't have (prenatal) genetic testing done." And, indeed, though figures are not available for reasons of personal privacy and confidentiality, it is certainly reasonable to believe that many couples who are confronted with pregnancies likely to lead to children with special needs choose to abort those pregnancies, even when those special needs can be managed fairly successfully.

We have elected not to discuss abortion as a health policy or health care ethics issue because attitudes about abortion are often reached and held in ways that do not reflect the kinds of ethical decision-making approaches we have advocated in this book. Abortion as an issue often triggers emotional and religious responses not conducive to mutual understanding or interpersonal solution. Nevertheless, the ethical problem of abortions due to genetic-test results cannot be ignored. Without attempting to address the larger issues surrounding abortion, we must recognize that deliberate abortion is never a trivial matter. Even unplanned pregnancies are invested with intense hopes, feelings, and fears. Moreover, abortion unavoidably ends a life that may have intrinsic value and almost certainly has the potential for the unique individual humanity that many consider to be a kind of ultimate value. No one who has ever undergone or assisted with an abortion can be entirely unaffected by the experience, and many are severely scarred by it. Whether or not abortion is ever ethically justifiable, it is never ethically unimportant.

Thus, people on all sides of the abortion controversy have strong reasons to do all they can to provide alternatives to abortion. Genetic testing prior to conceiving children can provide such an alternative because it allows prospective parents to decide in advance whether a genetic anomaly they are likely to pass on to their offspring is associated with a disease condition severe enough that it would be unloving or irresponsible to afflict their children with it. There are, after all, alternatives. Prospective parents can reconcile themselves to childlessness or to adopting children. Or, in some cases, genetic technology can already offer the opportunity to select and implant a healthy embryo rather than one afflicted with the genetic problem that will lead to disease.

Case 9.1: Prenatal Testing and Parental Responsibility

Joel and Rachael Kowalski have waited to have children until they were both well-established in careers that provide them with ample income and job security. As they are both in their late thirties, an age when the potential for "problem pregnancies" increases, their obstetrician recommends genetic testing prior to conception and further testing and monitoring during the pregnancy. As a result of preimplantation genetic screening, they discover that they both carry the gene for Tay-Sachs disease, which means that there is a 25 percent chance their child would be afflicted with the disease. Joel and Rachael very much want a child, but they do not want their child afflicted with Tay-Sachs disease; and they are hesitant to adopt because, as deeply religious Jews, they want a child of their own ethnicity. Their genetic counselor points out that they have options other than adoption. In vitro fertilization combined with embryonic testing will enable selection and implantation of an embryo that is free from the genetic anomaly that produces the disease.

Joel and Rachael are not at risk for developing Tay-Sachs disease themselves. And until recently, they would have gone ahead and had a child, accepting the results of the genetic lottery however they turned out. If their child had Tay-Sachs, the result would have been tragic for them and their child, but since nothing was available to help them to avoid or mitigate the problem, they would have been considered unfortunate rather than irresponsible in going ahead with the pregnancy. Now, however, they are in a position to avoid the problem altogether, though at considerable cost and by means that raise ethical problems. Many argue that in the new environment created by genetic technology, Joel and Rachael's moral responsibilities have changed. Does the existence of tests that can predict serious diseases create a moral responsibility in susceptible people to find out their risks and the risks they will pass on to their offspring? Does a positive result on a screening make prospective parents morally irresponsible if they bring a child with serious defects into the world when little or nothing can be done to give that child a reasonably normal life? Do such parents have a moral responsibility to do everything they can to avoid bearing a child whose life will be filled with great suffering? Would the Kowalskis be doing something irresponsible *not* to make use of preimplantation selection technology if they intend to have a child?

Some ethicists have argued that prospective parents do have an obligation to assess their genetic risk factors. Some go further still, arguing that prospective couples have an obligation to assess their genetic risk factors, so that prior to making a marital commitment, people will know whether their prospective partners have Huntington's disease, a predisposition to Alzheimer's, or genetic markers for breast cancer, for example—because such conditions will create heavy burdens of anxiety, expense, and care for the other spouse and family. Others have argued that, unless others are likely to be affected *very* seriously indeed, there ought to be a zone of privacy that protects individuals' unwillingness to be tested or to disclose the results of tests. There is also some question whether such distant—and, with scientific progress, perhaps avoidable—problems ought to have to be disclosed. Moreover, there are legitimate fears that the results of tests and disclosures may have troubling effects, ranging from depression, even suicide, in the face of severe conditions for which there are no effective therapies or cures to rejection or severe tensions in people's relationships to loss of employment and denial of health care insurance coverage. (We will discuss these last two issues later in the chapter.)

Does a positive result for a serious disease like Tay-Sachs mean that conceiving a child without taking steps to avoid the problem would be irresponsible, given that little or nothing can be done to provide a Tay-Sachs child with anything like a normal life? Some would argue that such a step would indeed be ethically irresponsible. One reason is that having genetically related children is hardly a human right that is to be exercised at all costs. However, while procreating may not be a human right that supersedes obligations to the rest of the human community, certainly bearing genetically related children is a human value that may conflict with other equally significant values.

Knowingly bearing a Tay-Sachs child means incurring immense costs, not only in terms of money, but also in terms of resources that cannot be used to address other needs and in terms of the strain on care providers. Perhaps more important, the child will suffer greatly without developing the capacities normally associated with good lives—lives full of joy and the potential for growth, development, and fulfillment. Here is one statement of this view:

> A principle of parental responsibility should require of individuals that they attempt to refrain from having children unless certain minimal conditions can be satisfied. This principle maintains that in deciding whether to have children, people should not be concerned only with their own interests in reproducing. They must think also, and perhaps primarily, of the welfare of the children they will bear. They should ask themselves "What kind of life is my child likely to have?" Individuals who will make good parents—that is, loving, concerned parents—will want their children to have lives well worth living and will strive to give them such lives. But what if the parents cannot give their children even a decent chance at a good life? The principle of parental responsibility maintains that under such conditions, it is better not to have children, and that it is in fact unfair to children to bring them into the world with "the deck stacked against them." (Steinbock and McClamrock, 1994, pp. 15–21)

But these lines of argument need hardly go unquestioned. It is hard to quarrel with the idea that prospective parents have a responsibility to think carefully about the welfare of the children they hope to bear. But it is far from obvious that in order to be valuable, human life must at least offer normal opportunities for good lives; nor is it obvious how to define what a good life is. One grave danger of the genetic revolution is what might be called "perfect baby syndrome," the idea that all babies must be entirely free of any special needs or anomalous limitations. Another comes from ignoring the unique contributions to value that handicapped individuals can make in their own lives and the lives of all the rest of humanity. And surely it is not obvious that a good life requires a greater balance of happiness than suffering.

There is no universal understanding or definition of a good life. Should there be?

Many people, some religious and some not, reject the idea that human lives have to "earn" value through development, relationship, and actions. Perhaps human lives have intrinsic value; perhaps their value is not conferred on them by their accomplishments or the investment made in them by others, but simply by being who they are. Perhaps human lives have value because a supreme being loves them; perhaps even lives filled with terrible suffering are redeemed by their relationship with a supreme being. Perhaps the resolution to provide a suffering child the most loving, supportive environment possible is not evidence of parental irresponsibility, but evidence of profound moral commitment of a kind beyond the imaginations of those who have not undertaken it. Perhaps even a brief experience of being loved is enough to say that a suffering child's life was not without profound value.

Do prospective parents with genetic anomalies have a responsibility to do *everything* they can to avoid bearing a child whose life will be filled with great suffering due to receiving a genetic endowment that includes those anomalies? Here the answer must be "certainly not." Such a sweeping requirement is far too restrictive. Since not all genetic anomalies can be detected or anticipated (some, after all, occur spontaneously), this would require either celibacy, which would prevent the bearing of children with any risk of genetic abnormality, or abortion, which would prevent any genetically abnormal child from being born—neither of which is remotely acceptable. But many ethicists have argued that parents have a responsibility to go to great lengths to avoid bearing children whose lives are filled with suffering. Would the Kowalskis be doing something irresponsible by not taking advantage of selective in vitro fertilization and implantation?

PREIMPLANTATION GENETIC TECHNOLOGY

The technology offered to the Kowalskis involves taking a number of ova from Rachael and fertilizing them in vitro with sperm taken from Joel. Multiple conceptions will occur, each of which is then allowed to grow to at least an eight-celled stage, when they can be genetically analyzed. Some of these embryos will have two copies of the Tay-Sachs gene; if one of those embryos were implanted and born, the child would develop the disease. Some will have only one copy of the gene, which means they would develop into carriers, but not suffer the disease. Some embryos will be free of the Tay-Sachs gene, which means that those children would neither experience the disease nor carry it. Joel and Rachael would like Tay-Sachs-free embryos implanted. They recognize that the fertilization and implantation process may have to be done a number of times before the implantation "takes" and Rachael's pregnancy can continue normally. Is there anything ethically problematic about this?

> *In vitro fertilization (IVF) technology has provided hope for many couples with fertility problems. It involves the use of strong hormones to stimulate the production of many ova in the female parent, and these are then retrieved through endoscopic surgery. The ova are then fertilized with sperm from the male parent and incubated. At precisely the right time interval, the embryos are then implanted, also by endoscopic surgery. Timing is critical because all the steps involved must mimic the biological process. Although a few states have required insurers to cover IVF, in most states these procedures are not a covered insurance benefit and the couple must pay for the procedures, which may cost approximately $10,000 for each trial. There are no guarantees that the cycle of procedures performed will result in pregnancy. Indeed, there are couples who participate in IVF more than once.*

As we observed earlier, abortion is never an ethically trivial matter, and some will see the procedure as involving a number of abortions. Those who believe that "life begins at conception"—that from the moment of conception embryos are fully human persons who deserve the same moral standing as any other persons—will object that when those "defective" embryos not implanted are discarded, they are, in effect, murdered, just as "unborn children" are murdered by abortions further along in the process of their development. From this perspective, it does not matter that those embryos cannot suffer because they lack the neurological network that is physiologically required for suffering. It also does not matter that a great deal of suffering is being prevented by the discarding of these embryos. From this point of view, destroying defective embryos is simply and absolutely wrong, and no number of beneficial results can outweigh the wrongness of such killing.[1]

---

[1] It is not easy to do real justice to this position, often associated with the right-to-life movement. Those who do not share the conviction that embryos are persons in the full moral sense from the moment of conception often ask what it is about embryos that makes them sufficiently similar to persons to make it reasonable to attribute full moral status to them. To ask this question is to miss the essential point of the "conceptionist" position, which is that being a person with full moral status is not something that human offspring have to earn at any stage of their development; it is something they *are* simply by being themselves. Not being able to see this is regarded by conceptionists as blameworthy moral blindness on a par with being unable to understand what was so bad about the Holocaust. Being asked to defend the wrongness of abortion in terms of other interests sacrificed, larger social issues, or rights which outweigh other rights places conceptionists in a false position because the wrongness of abortion is seen as morally more basic, fundamental, and absolute than other interests, issues, or rights. Their inability to reply in terms familiar to those who reason according to utilitarian principles of balancing interests, for example, makes conceptionists appear unreasonable, while those who ask for explanations about what is wrong with abortion seem, to conceptionists, morally depraved.

Moreover, the use of this technology to select for and against desired traits raises other questions. Even those who can accept its use to avoid Tay-Sachs disease might be less comfortable selecting against embryos with less serious genetic anomalies. Would it make any difference to our ethical judgments if the condition being selected against were something like Down's Syndrome, a condition that permits a full and rich, if not entirely normal life? Should (prospective) parents be permitted to select against dwarf embryos?[2] Or in favor of one sex or the other? Or against embryos genetically prone to manic depression or late-onset Alzheimer's? Or against offspring prone to obesity? Or, ultimately, as testing becomes ever more detailed, should (prospective) parents be morally permitted to select in favor of desired hair color, height, and personality traits?

Prospects like these seem to many too much like *Brave New World,* too fraught with dangers of abuse and discrimination to be morally tolerable. Some fear that such genetic manipulation would lead to a genetic uniformity of humanity that would threaten the very real values of diversity and pluralism, in effect creating a society of Barbies and Kens, every one of whom would be, in Garrison Keillor's phrase, "above average."

Of course, the prospect of cloning technology raises similar concerns: that human individuality will be lost and the unique value of every person will be undermined. But there are good reasons to think that these fears may be much exaggerated. Identical twins have the same genetic endowment, but they are hardly identical persons without distinctive individuality. Besides, even if responsible parents would not wish to inflict painful diseases on their children, and even if there is substantial agreement on what counts as a disease, there is, fortunately, much less agreement on what are the most desirable traits in one's own children. As one of our Hispanic students pointed out, "Why would I want my daughter to look like Barbie?"

SOCIAL AND ECONOMIC CONSIDERATIONS

The issue of how much control parents ought to be able to exert in selecting the genetic endowments of their children is an important and unsettling one. Another reason it is ethically troubling is that many people who have conditions prospective parents tend to select against feel demeaned by the fact that they are selected against and fear that if selection against dwarfism, say, becomes widespread, those dwarves who

---

[2] Again, the point of the conceptionist position is that those who make use of in vitro fertilization are *prospective* parents only up to the moment their ova and sperm are united; from that moment on they are parents.

remain will be subjected to even more abusive discrimination. There is, perhaps, also reason to fear that as preimplantation technology becomes more widely available and more commonly used, those who have children with genetically based diseases will no longer be regarded as unfortunate, but rather as irresponsible. Perhaps societal attitudes toward those parents or, worse, toward their children will become even more unsympathetic and intolerant.

> *Until genetic technology made it possible to change the outcomes of genetic heredity, our human community accepted the outcome of the genetic lottery as a part of the risks inherent in being alive. The human community established health care (or disease care) as a social institution for the common good. What do these ideas of genetic engineering imply for our social institutions?*

It is also a short step from this attitude to an economic argument along the following lines. Since the parents of "defective" children made the choice to assume the burdens of childbearing under these difficult conditions, they can hardly expect others to share the load. Thus, some have argued, parents who elect not to avoid the expensive consequences of having children with special needs can expect to pay for them themselves. Such an argument might be used to oppose special education funding, for example, or handicapped services, or even to modify existing antidiscrimination statutes.

These lines of argument can certainly be challenged. First, not all genetically based disease conditions can be tested for or identified prior to birth, so it would clearly be wrong to hold people blameworthy for failing to anticipate and prevent them; furthermore, markers can be misidentified or not disclosed through errors in testing. Second, this line of argument will certainly lead to intense pressure (amounting to coercion) on many people to abort their pregnancies. No parties to the abortion controversy have ever maintained that anyone ought to be compelled to abort a pregnancy; the most that has ever been seriously argued is that people ought to have the legal and moral right to abort if they choose to do so.

Third, these lines of argument suggest a degree of individual responsibility that is genuinely cruel, supportable only by those, one suspects, who are pretty sure they are and will always remain among the (genetically) fortunate. And fourth, they beg important questions about what makes lives valuable.

Yet discrimination against people with genetic anomalies is already occurring. One unintended result of genetic testing is the release of results to one's employer and one's insurance company. For a time, the U.S. Department of Defense excluded people with sickle cell genes from admission to the Air Force Academy—even those with one copy of the normal allele and one copy of the sickling allele who will never develop the disease, although there was no evidence that they were in any way more susceptible to health problems than anyone else.[3] People who have tested positive for Huntington's disease have lost their employment when their susceptibilities came to the attention of their employers, often, apparently, because employers are reluctant to shoulder the financial burdens of more expensive health insurance and disability. Insurance companies have used the results of genetic testing to exclude benefits for conditions now regarded as "preexisting" and also to raise the rates of people likely to incur higher-than-normal costs due to genetic anomalies.

At this writing, genetic testing is an almost entirely voluntary matter. That is, although some physicians might recommend submitting to testing because of pregnancy, family history, or the precursors of disease, it is still relatively easy for those who are unwilling to undergo testing or who do not want to know their disease propensities to simply refuse. The reluctance of many people to be tested is easily understandable in the many cases where there are neither cures nor effective therapies. Testing positive for one of these conditions can amount to a death sentence, prompting despair, and it has led to profound depression and even suicide in some cases. It has also led to some extremely dubious measures, such as removing the breasts and uterus of a young woman with an 80 percent chance of having breast cancer or ovarian cancer by age 65. However, testing can enable people to anticipate and perhaps prevent problems, thus avoiding more expensive treatment later on.

Considerations of expense and loss of employee services may incline more employers and insurance companies to make genetic screening a precondition for employment or coverage; and then genetic testing becomes far less a personal, voluntary matter. The argument is that neither private employers nor private insurance companies are social welfare agencies; their role is to generate profits for their owners and stockholders by providing goods and services at competitive prices. Such an argument will make sense to those unwilling to subsidize other people's risks. Many companies now have a policy not to hire cigarette smokers because they typically experience far more illness and incur higher health care costs than do nonsmokers; many insurance companies similarly will not insure smokers or insure them at substantially higher rates for the same reasons. They find it difficult to see any relevant

---

[3] This example is cited by Philip Kitcher in *The Lives to Come* (New York: Simon and Schuster, 1996), p. 130.

difference between the case of cigarette smokers whose smoking gives them a predisposition to heart and lung diseases and the case of someone who has a predisposition to those or other debilitating conditions because of genetic anomalies.

It is tempting to reply that smoking is voluntary while genetic heritage is not, so that discriminating against smokers in hiring is not morally offensive in the way that discriminating against those susceptible to conditions over which they have no control is. However, emerging genetic technology and changing public attitudes about responsibility make this answer less obviously persuasive to some. First, it appears that the propensity to find smoking almost irresistibly satisfying and to become addicted to it both physically and psychologically has a genetic basis. But, more important, there appears to be an increasing disinclination on the part of many people to accept any responsibility for other people's misfortunes. Individualism, originating with our Puritan roots, suggests that each person has the potential to succeed or fail as the result of his or her own efforts. Evolution of individualism further suggests that our failures are our own responsibility. This understanding is the basis for "blaming the victim" and has been used to justify ignoring unpopular disease conditions.

Even though the circumstances that plunge many people into poverty are often matters over which they have little or no control, the public at large seems less and less willing to share in supporting them through welfare and other programs; the indigent are expected to take responsibility for themselves. Similarly, even though the circumstances that leave many people with serious disease conditions and other handicaps may be entirely beyond their control, there appears to be an increasing tendency to expect that they should deal with their misfortunes without expecting others to shoulder any of the costs. Why, they ask, should our group premiums go up and up to provide benefits to someone we know in advance will eventually incur very costly care? Why not simply avoid the problem by employing and insuring only those with normal, comparable risks?

If testing becomes widespread and the results are used to determine employment and insurance, many people with genetic anomalies will find themselves marginalized by society. Clearly that is unfortunate for them; is it also morally wrong? Many ethicists would argue that it is. Health, and access to health care, is not a consumer product in the ordinary sense; it is a precondition for being able to lead anything like a normal life. And fair access to employment opportunities seems to be a similarly necessary condition for leading a normal life. In both cases, to deprive people of such fundamental goods without compelling, morally justifiable reasons seems thoroughly unjust. That employers and insurance companies are eager to minimize their costs and maximize their profits and that consumers want the prices they pay for goods and services, including insurance premiums, to be cut do not seem to provide morally compelling reasons to deprive a number of unlucky people of fundamentally important opportunities for health care and employment.

Making a comparison between voluntarily choosing to smoke and a genetic predisposition to cancer in order to allow higher premiums in both cases is arguably false. As Philip Kitcher points out, "perhaps higher premiums for health insurance are justified when the applicants have voluntarily overindulged all the wrong habits, knowing the medical effects—although the fashionable war on tobacco, alcohol, and fatty foods might itself be charged with Puritanical excess." But if a woman is born with a genetic predisposition to some form of cancer, there is nothing she did or could do that would reduce her risks to a level similar to those of people without her genetic endowment. "If, no matter what she had done, she would still have been at higher risk, then the duty to protect her against loss of a fundamental resource, the ability to maintain her health, cannot be canceled by holding her responsible" (Kitcher, 1996, pp. 134–35). And surely it would be even more unjust to hold her responsible— by forcing her to pay much higher premiums, for example—for her parents' failure to have made different reproductive choices or perhaps to have aborted her.

Here is one more social and economic problem with genetic screening and technology. Though individual tests are not extremely expensive relative to other medical procedures, they can be well beyond the ability to pay of many people, many of them Americans, and more in the Third World. Even further out of reach is access to the kinds of preimplantation screening and in vitro fertilization available to the Kowalskis, which, at this writing, would cost in the range of $30,000. Given the serious problems with access to even a minimally adequate level of health care services in the United States and many other places, how high a priority should be given to assuring access to genetic technologies? Is it unjust that many people will not be able to make use of these services? (It would certainly be unjust to hold them in any way responsible for genetic choices without giving them access to genetic services.)

Answers to these questions are deeply connected to how we view reproduction, the well-being of children, and our collective responsibilities to promote healthy families, as well as our views of access to health care generally. Neither individual nor societal resources are infinite, and extending a full range of genetic services to everyone would be extremely costly. Yet it seems morally reprehensible that we permit such gross inequities in access to such fundamental goods as prenatal services. And it also seems morally reprehensible that we deprive parents of the means to prevent serious suffering on the part of children whose lives will be blighted by the most serious genetic disorders. Unfortunately, no solution immediately presents itself.[4]

QUESTIONS FOR DISCUSSION

1. *Case 9.2: Genetic Knowledge and Responsibility*—Arlo's father died of Huntington's disease, which means that Arlo has a 50 percent chance of developing it himself. All other things being equal, any children Arlo might have will have a 25 percent likelihood of developing Huntington's disease. With which of the following statements do you agree? What reasons do you have for your decisions in each case?

   a. Arlo is under no obligation to find out whether he has the genetic endowment for Huntington's disease.

   b. Arlo has a moral obligation to inform his fiancée of the probability that he will develop Huntington's disease and that it can be passed on to their children—before they marry or have children.

   c. If Arlo and his wife find out that the fetus she is carrying has the Huntington's gene, and they are not morally opposed to abortion, they should abort this pregnancy.

   d. Knowing their risks, Arlo and his wife should make use of selective in vitro fertilization to avoid having children with Huntington's disease.

2. Assuming that selective in vitro fertilization is at least sometimes morally acceptable, and assuming that it would be possible in each case, which conditions do you think can legitimately be selected for or against? In each case, why? Within a few years, it should become possible to modify the genes responsible for these and other conditions in desired directions. Which of these conditions

---

[4] Throughout this section, and for many of the questions that follow, we are deeply indebted to participants in the Genome Technology & Reproduction: Values and Public Policy project, sponsored by the National Institutes of Health through the University of Michigan Council on Genetics & Society and the Michigan State University Center for Ethics & Humanities in the Life Sciences. Particular thanks go to Professor Leonard Fleck of MSU, many of whose ideas appear in this section in various guises.

do you think ought to be permitted to be modified in the desired direction? How and why, if at all, are your answers different from the question about selection?

a. Tay-Sachs disease

b. Down's syndrome

c. Dwarfism

d. Bipolar disorder (manic-depressive disorder)

e. Homosexuality

f. Male-pattern baldness

g. Female-pattern baldness

h. Being female

3. Should comprehensive genetic screening and counseling become the routine standard of care for prospective parents? For people generally? Who should have access to the results of such tests (whether or not they become routine)? Should employment or insurance rate decisions be influenced by this kind of information? Why or why not?

CHAPTER TEN

Confidentiality, Patients, and Staff

TYPICAL CONFIDENTIALITY PROBLEMS

The obligation to preserve patient confidentiality has a long-standing basis in health care ethics. For example, it is specifically mentioned as part of the Hippocratic oath, which states that "What I see or hear in the course of the treatment . . . which on no account one must spread about, I will keep to myself." And this traditional commitment appears to be upheld by the mission statements, patients' rights documents, and disciplinary practices of most of today's health care institutions. Here are two recent examples.

Case 10.1: Breach of Confidentiality Because of Carelessness

Lisa P. is a nursing student, assigned for clinical experience to a medical surgical unit. She spent most of the morning with a patient, Mr. Jonas, whose condition was serious and complicated, but who was also very friendly and cooperative with Lisa and her clinical supervisor. When lunch time came, Lisa met her friend Amanda in the elevator, and both excitedly compared notes about their patients. Unfortunately for Lisa, Mrs. Jonas, her patient's wife, was also in the elevator and was upset that Lisa was breaching confidentiality in this way; she reported Lisa to the clinical supervisor. As a result, Lisa was expelled from the nursing program.[1]

Case 10.2: Breach of Confidentiality to Protect Others' Welfare

LaVon is a member of the environmental services department responsible for preparing operating rooms for surgical cases. His friend Marie is

---

[1] This case is modified from a case presented in *Nursing 97*, October, in a column called "Legal Questions."

a surgical technician who has just finished working with the rest of the surgical team on a patient who has hepatitis B. As LaVon was about to enter the operating room, Marie warned him of the potential for personal exposure to communicable disease, a warning LaVon much appreciated. In fact, he wondered why warnings of potential for exposure were not standard policy, since he knew that nurses and surgeons often reminded each other when special precautions were needed. So LaVon wrote the hospital CEO as well as a number of other members of the administration describing the case, praising Marie, and demanding that environmental services be informed whenever a patient presented a potential for exposure to a communicable disease. Both LaVon and Marie received disciplinary action involving one-week suspensions without pay.

> Before going on, think about cases 10.1 and 10.2. Why exactly was what they did unprofessional? Do you think Lisa, La Von, and Marie were disciplined appropriately? How would you have handled their situations?

Cases like these suggest that patients and their families expect confidentiality to be preserved and that health care organizations can be aggressive in disciplining staff members who violate confidentiality, particularly in ways that embarrass their colleagues and institutions. Yet health care organizations can also be insensitive and lax in protecting patient confidentiality. Consider this case.

Case 10.3: Routine Breaches of Confidentiality

Eldon G. is a successful businessman, but he is suffering sexual dysfunction. He suspects that his high-stress work life is making him impotent. He crosses the waiting room at Health Plus Clinic, which is full of women and children, approaches the desk, and signs in. As he turns back to find a seat, the receptionist asks, "What will you be seeing doctor for, Mr. G.?" Quiet chuckles and looks follow his answer. When he is admitted, he walks down the hall and notices all the patient charts and records hanging on the doors to the examining rooms. Recognizing the name of a business associate, he notices the word "hemorrhoids." After half an hour, during which time Eldon could not help but overhear the stern "lose weight" lecture someone named Elaine was getting in the next room, a new physician's assistant, Diane M., entered the exam room without knocking ("I'm glad I wasn't undressed," Eldon thought). As Elaine walked by the open examining room door, Diane said, "OK, Eldon, I see you're having problems with impotence. By the way, are you by any chance Robin's husband? Robin and I are in a step aerobics class together."

It takes little imagination to see that Eldon's privacy has been thoroughly compromised in this situation and that he is almost certainly experiencing profound embarrassment. Imagine how he will feel once he starts receiving pharmaceutical offers and mail-order marital aid ads in the mail, since, like many other physicians' groups and pharmacists, the Health Plus Clinic allows a data collection group to buy information about patients that is then resold to marketing departments for targeted mailings. Nothing in this case suggests any intentional violations of confidentiality. But the result is deeply troubling to those concerned about patient privacy.

Part of the problem about patient confidentiality is a conflict between traditional expectations concerning confidentiality and the way health care is delivered in our contemporary society. Health care professionals have traditionally been expected to maintain confidentiality, and patients have traditionally taken this for granted. But this traditional concept of confidentiality is based on a form of health care delivery that is no longer common. Rather, it is based on the model which assumes that there is one physician, and perhaps one nurse, to whom patients disclose sensitive information about themselves and that no one else has either a legitimate claim to this information or would discover it in the normal course of health care delivery. In the current environment of health care, these assumptions are, of course, thoroughly misplaced.

In normal hospitalizations, for example, dozens of physicians, nurses, medical and nursing technologists of many kinds, discharge planners, and many other clinical personnel will normally come into contact with sensitive patient information. So will dozens of clerical, finance, and insurance personnel. And this list does not even mention the many others who may give themselves access to such information accidentally or in other ways unrelated to legitimate patient services.

> It is common for the average medical record to be seen by dozens of people. The People's Medical Society (1996) reported, "The typical paper medical record is viewed by as many as 77 different people during the average hospital stay." Considering the accessibility of electronic records, this total may rise.

As a practical matter, preserving confidentiality is much more difficult than ever before and may even be a hopeless task. In this environment, what is confidentiality, why should health care providers care about respecting patient confidentiality, and what should they do to preserve it?

WHAT IS CONFIDENTIALITY?

One reasonable definition of confidentiality, at least as the idea plays out in a contemporary health care setting, is control over information. Preserving confidentiality is providing information and access to information only to those specifically authorized by the patient or to those who require the information in order to perform services specifically authorized by the patient. This definition means that patients do not have to be consulted each and every time someone has access to information about them. However, they do need to be made aware of who will have access and why, so their informed consent can be granted (or refused). It also means that, if confidentiality is to be respected, subsequent access to patient information should be limited to those who really do need it in order to perform services the patient authorizes.

> *Privacy is a value closely related to confidentiality, but it covers much more ground. Whereas* confidentiality *concerns access to and control over information,* privacy *concerns the whole range of activities people engage in with a reasonable expectation that they will not be subjected to the view, presence, intrusion, or interference of others.*

Breaches of confidentiality can occur for reasons that are well-meaning, such as when Smith asks Jones's advice about what to do in Mrs. Brown's case. They can occur through inattention, when a group of nurses gets used to chatting about their patients over lunch and others not involved in their care take an interest in the conversation, or in cases like Lisa and Amanda's, where the patient's wife overhears an inappropriate but common conversation. They can occur through thoughtlessness, such as when charts are left where they can easily be seen (as in the case of Eldon G. at the Health Plus Clinic). These breaches can occur through insensitive institutional arrangements, as when a case presenting an interesting pathology is used for continuing education without a competent patient's permission or when charts are left in plain view. Or breaches can occur intentionally as when a staff member warns another staff member that a patient is HIV-positive or has another infectious disease condition, so that special precautions can be taken (the case of LaVon and Marie).

What, exactly, is so bad about violating confidentiality? Sometimes, violating patient confidentiality has no very serious adverse consequences, at least on the surface. But, sometimes, it can have far-reaching effects: the breakup of a marriage, a job dismissal, discrimination, or denial of insurance coverage or benefits. These harms, whether material or emotional or both, are real and important reasons not to violate confidentiality. But they are not the only reasons. Even if we as individuals know that "nothing is going to come of it" and "nobody is going to care," it would still be professionally irresponsible and unethical for health care providers to violate confidentiality.

Confiding in an individual means entrusting personal knowledge. Health care providers are then privileged to know all our health secrets along with understanding the seemingly mysterious processes of the human body. Health care providers become our health "confessors," those to whom we bare our physical and emotional selves.

Another important reason to respect confidentiality is that patients are often embarrassed or uncomfortable about their conditions. But, for care to be effective, patients must disclose these uncomfortable aspects of their situations to health care providers. If patients fear that embarrassing or uncomfortable information may be passed to others, many will be shamed and humiliated enough not to reveal that information in the first place. This has been a particular problem with sexually transmissible diseases, HIV-positive status, and other health problems carrying social stigma. Patients with these conditions who have been unable or unwilling to trust that their confidentiality will be preserved have simply concealed these conditions from care providers. When that happens, their care is compromised, their chances for recovering health will be diminished, and others, including health care personnel, are placed at serious risk. Preserving confidentiality promotes an atmosphere of trust that is absolutely essential for effective care and cooperative patients. Violating it produces distrust and noncompliant patients. So confidentiality has to be maintained.

But what about a situation in which a care provider violates confidentiality because she thinks that doing so would benefit the patient— would get her to face up to abuse problems in her marriage, say, or to deal with her substance abuse problem—or would guide the care provider in giving better service? There's a simple and effective alternative to violating confidentiality in those situations: get the patient's permission first. But if that is impossible or inconvenient, it would still normally be unprofessional to violate the patient's confidentiality, even to benefit the patient. It is a violation of the patient's fundamental human dignity. To see why, though, takes us deeper into some of the most basic of human values.

THE DEEP VALUE OF CONFIDENTIALITY

What is the real value of confidentiality? More broadly, why is respecting privacy important? Who we are as unique individuals is very much bound up with the network of relationships we have with others. Our spouses, our family members, and our closest friends are at the heart of this network. These are people we not only feel we can share our deepest thoughts and feelings with, but they are also people we are confident will care about those thoughts and feelings in the right way. Sharing information that touches the core of our being exposes us and makes us vulnerable, but we do share private information with people we feel know, understand, and love us (despite ourselves). Sharing our deepest thoughts and feelings makes people vulnerable because those thoughts and feelings are close to the core of who we are as persons. One irony is that we must have confidence in others in order to have confidence in ourselves. Self-confidence and self-worth are necessary ingredients for being a healthy person. We need the love and understanding of those closest to us, and we can be deeply wounded by their neglect, ridicule, or rejection. So we carefully control how much, and what, we reveal about ourselves even to those we trust the most. That sense of control over how far we let people in is an important element of our sense of who we are as persons.

Moreover, the full, rich network of human relationships that are part of people's lives is truly impossible without a reasonable level of privacy and confidentiality. In some respects, intimacy is a matter of how deeply we know those with whom we have relationships. There are things that a spouse, for example, or a lover needs to know that others, such as business associates or tennis partners or employers not only do not need to know, but also would be much better off not knowing. If we share personal matters with someone who is not in the right sort of relationship to know these matters, we place a strain on the existing relationship and pressure others to be closer or more intimate than they might be comfortable with.

When we are forced to reveal personal information about ourselves to strangers, we usually attempt to provide the barest minimum necessary to get something done—to take out a mortgage, for example, or to get admitted to a hospital. Even then we often resent some of the questions we may have to answer ("What business is it of theirs what my mother's maiden name was?" we might ask). When someone uses the information we provide in a way we would not have authorized, we have lost control over our lives and are at the mercy of people we do not know. If information about ourselves that makes us feel vulnerable or humiliated is passed on without our consent, trust is lost and we may fear being treated disrespectfully. In fact, we may feel violated even when information about us is not misused, if that information is sufficiently embarrassing or if the potential for embarrassment is sufficiently great.

Further, when confidentiality is broken, we have been violated and wronged even when we are unaware of it. If Eldon G.'s employees or business associates hear about his sexual dysfunction, he may well become the source of jokes at his expense. Whether he ever hears them or not, those jokes will change the attitude that others will adopt toward him in ways almost certain to work against his interests. The situation may even be far worse with a sexually transmissible disease or HIV-positive status. A patient might not know that his condition has been divulged, but people's attitudes and behavior toward him, even among health care providers, will certainly change, again in detrimental ways. So we need to respect patient confidentiality. Even when there is no material harm, even when people are unaware that their privacy has been breached, violating confidentiality is a deep affront to people's dignity. As the possessors of intimate, personal details about people, we need to uphold the trust they put in us and not reveal information to anyone they would not authorize.

THE LIMITS OF CONFIDENTIALITY

But is this obligation absolute? Are there ever circumstances when breaching confidentiality is professionally responsible? Yes, there are. We are required by law to report suspected instances of child or elder abuse or neglect (in some states, spouse abuse as well), gunshot wounds, and some communicable diseases. Of course, the fact that these are legal obligations does not by itself make them ethical obligations. But there are also strong ethical reasons to report child or elder abuse—namely to protect the interests of those persons who are otherwise likely to be vulnerable or helpless. There are ethical reasons to report gunshot wounds, since the interests of society in safety and security arguably outweigh the privacy interests of individuals. And there are ethical reasons to report some communicable diseases, having to do with protecting important public health values and providing innocent third parties with the opportunity to protect themselves from serious injury and disease. (Often this can be done by using identification other than names of patients to preserve confidentiality.) Moreover, since these laws are, at least in theory, public knowledge, patients who seek medical services can be expected to know that information about these matters will be disclosed. Of course, patients may not know this or may assume that disclosure is entirely at the provider's discretion. Such patients need and deserve to be told about providers' obligations in these regards. They may not accept the situation with any degree of comfort. But this kind of disclosure is not an unprofessional violation of confidentiality; in fact, it would be unprofessional in most cases of these kinds *not* to disclose.

More difficult are situations in which there is no legal duty to disclose information, but others besides the patient are threatened or at risk. A famous case is one in which a psychologist learned from a patient of the patient's intent to murder a former girlfriend. The case raised two questions: Was there enough evidence here to inform the police (which the psychologist did)? And was there an obligation to tell the young woman or her family (which was not done)? The consensus among ethicists is that the young woman ought to have been informed. This is because the serious harm threatened to her was sufficient to override the professional duty to preserve confidentiality, and there seemed to be no way to avoid the threat while preserving confidentiality. But it is important to note that *both* conditions need to be met for overriding confidentiality, not just the threat of harm alone. If there had been a way to preserve confidentiality while protecting those under threat, that resolution would have been preferable to protecting them by violating patient confidentiality, at least from the point of view of health care ethics. Therefore, to override confidentiality in cases like these requires two things: a credible threat of serious harm and no practical way to prevent that harm without violating confidentiality.

So what about cases in which those who are threatened with harm are friends, coworkers, or colleagues? Imagine that a patient has a dangerous, highly infectious disease, such as some forms of hepatitis, or perhaps a dangerous but only moderately infectious disease, such as AIDS. Although the actual risk of transmission from patients to hospital staff is minimal, especially when practice is careful and conscientious, the consequences of infection could be catastrophic for a person who became infected.[2] Does that give health professionals the right to violate patient confidentiality by informing each other that a specific patient is haz-

---

[2] No reliable information appears to exist on how many health care workers have been infected with blood-borne diseases while they were observing universal precautions. (Blood is the only body fluid implicated in occupational transmission of HIV.) Accidental needle stick injury is the most common form of exposure to blood, and current estimates are that 800,000 accidental needle sticks occur each year (Stark, 1993). There is a 0.3 percent to 0.4 percent risk of infection for each needle stick event. However, over 50 percent of these needle sticks are caused by unnecessary needles, such as those sometimes still used to access intravenous equipment. Most of the rest are due to practice errors. "The most important instruction to health care workers that can reduce this risk is the following: do not recap needles. Other risk reduction measures include the adoption of universal precautions against transmission of infectious disease; sharp instrument precautions; the use of protective garb to prevent skin and mucous membrane contamination when blood or bloody body fluid may splash; the availability of stable, puncture resistant disposal containers for sharp instruments; the exclusion of breakable glass syringes; and the accessibility of resuscitation equipment in all rooms in order to avoid direct mouth to mouth contact" (Wall, Olcott, & Gererding, 1991).

ardous? Was what Marie did, warning a colleague of the danger of infection, really so bad? Would health care workers not have a right, maybe even a responsibility, to warn each other in order to preserve a safe working environment?

The short answer is still "No," except in certain emergency situations. This is because the important value of safeguarding staff normally can be accomplished without sacrificing the value of patient confidentiality. The standard of care that has been developed precisely to safeguard staff is to observe universal precautions, treating every patient as potentially infectious. "Universal precautions" is a general term for wearing gloves, masks, and gowns sufficient to protect people from contaminants without first verifying whether a patient has any disease condition that places people at risk. While observing such precautions can be expensive, time-consuming, and tiresome—and, to some patients, can even seem offensive—the practice of universal precautions accomplishes the best outcome from the point of view of health care ethics, sacrificing only some values of comfort and convenience for providers while preserving the most important values of safeguarding staff safety and also preserving patient confidentiality.

Moreover, from a staff safety point of view, universal precautions offers another extremely important advantage. It offers the best possible protection against *undiagnosed* infectious conditions. This is because, if staff come to rely on warning signals to practice universal precautions conscientiously, they will be vulnerable whenever those warnings are not given. And warnings *won't* be given in cases in which staff don't know about a risk. Treating every case as if it were dangerously infectious is the only way to maximize staff safety. And it doesn't require a breach of confidentiality to do so.

Prior to the advent of universal precautions, it was commonplace to delineate patient "isolation" procedures by door placards that carefully outlined all the steps to be taken to reduce exposure. Universal precautions eliminated that practice. However, now that there are antibiotic-resistant organisms present in our world, new isolation precautions are evolving. Rooms with negative pressure are required for patients who may have tuberculosis. And special door placards have been used to identify methicillin-resistant Staphylococcus aureus (MRSA). Do these practices violate confidentiality?

But what about a situation in which a staff member who is not observing universal precautions is about to be exposed to contaminated or infectious materials? Here there seem to be two kinds of cases. One case can be addressed by reminding the staff member to observe universal precautions, something that can be done without violating confidentiality even if "everyone knows" why the reminder is being given.

But the other kind of case would be one in which there is no time or opportunity to warn a colleague in any other way. Such a case would be extremely rare. Yelling "Stop" would almost always be as effective as yelling "Stop! He's got HIV!" But if there were such a situation, it would almost certainly be an "emergency" for which an exception would be justified. If there is no other practical way to safeguard a colleague than to violate confidentiality, and the risk is serious, as HIV contamination certainly would be, then the violation (the warning) would be ethically acceptable. But there are almost always other, better ways to give a warning that do protect confidentiality.

> *Universal precautions, if practiced as it was intended, would actually work. But health care providers sometimes forget to practice it or begin to take shortcuts to save valuable time. In life-threatening situations, it sometimes seems irresponsible to take the few minutes to don protective attire.*

Health care professionals face many stressful situations in the course of their practices. Sometimes patient confidentiality gets lost in casual conversations or through other inadvertent means. Moreover, the fragmentation and specialization of service delivery in contemporary health care spreads patient information to many people unknown to the patients, including many who are well outside the circle of care providers. Nevertheless, the value of confidentiality is indispensable if we are to respect our patients as persons and treat them with appropriate regard for human dignity. And it is indispensable also if we are to expect from our patients that they will willingly provide us with the information we need to serve their health care needs in a professionally responsible way. While there are a few problem cases in which patient confidentiality can be overridden, respecting patient confidentiality continues to be one of the most important obligations we have as ethical health care providers.

QUESTIONS FOR DISCUSSION

1. Return once more to the cases at the beginning of this chapter. What, exactly, was unprofessional about Lisa's, LaVon's, and Marie's behavior? Suppose that you were counseling them individually as a follow-up to these incidents. How would you explain "What's so bad about what I did?"

2. Thinking about Eldon G.'s case, what violations of patient confidentiality have you observed, either in your own use of health care services or in your workplace? What could be done to reduce or eliminate those violations?

3. How would you reply to staff who said this: "Why don't we warn each other about HIV patients? Wouldn't you like to know if it was your life at stake? Everybody says universal precautions, like they were some kind of magic formula. But they're time-consuming and uncomfortable, and anyway we have to know whether we're watching out for blood or TB. Gowns leak, gloves rip, people are human, accidents happen. The patients don't have to know we know. So what's the big deal?"

CONFIDENTIALITY AND PRIVACY AMONG COLLEAGUES

So far, we have discussed only one form of confidentiality, the duty health care providers have to respect the confidentiality of patients. However, there are other ethical issues involving confidentiality, two of which are especially important and common: confidentiality issues between health managers and the employees they manage, and confidentiality issues among members of the health care team. While employers certainly do have a legitimate need to know a good deal of information about their employees, there is also a sphere of privacy that employees legitimately expect to be recognized. Ethical conflicts can arise in drawing lines appropriately. Moreover, hospitals and other health care institutions are often hotbeds of gossip. Much of this gossip is probably harmless, but some of it can damage people's reputations or even careers. And there is also a potential for ethical conflict when an employee observes or believes that another health care professional has committed or is committing irresponsible or even unlawful acts. Confronting such people is always difficult. More difficult still would be a decision to "go public" or engage in what is called "whistle-blowing."

Case 10.4: Employee Confidentiality Versus Substance Abuse Problems

Although Saint Catherine's has instituted coded, locked cabinets for access to medications, it still has experienced episodes of medication diversion (medicines missing but unexplained), primarily of narcotics. Accordingly, it has instituted random drug screenings and spot checks of staff lockers, and it has mounted video monitors to oversee distribution sites. This morning, Angie B.'s nursing manager, Thom W., has taken her aside for a drug screen and locker check. In addition to the acute embarrassment of having to provide a urine sample under Thom's observation, Angie, who recently received a commendation from Thom for having completed a smoking cessation program, has just started smoking again and would really not like Thom to find the pack of cigarettes she has left in her jacket. Not wanting to be humiliated, Angie would refuse if she could. But she knows she can be suspended or fired for noncompliance with the policy, and she needs her job. What should Angie do?

Angie's situation is certainly uncomfortable, but it is also extremely common. The ethical issue here, as always, is one of balancing competing interests, specifically Angie's legitimate privacy interests against the interests of all the other parties involved. Her employer does have a legitimate interest in preventing theft and in safeguarding patients by assuring that no staff members are impaired by drug use. Saint Catherine's may also have an interest in maintaining the health of its staff by discouraging their smoking and use of illegal drugs. Moreover, courts have upheld drug testing to ensure the health and safety of workers and the public, even in cases where there is no "reasonable suspicion" of any particular person. Courts have been especially willing to sanction random or universal tests of those who may face emergency situations (nurses and police officers) or operate potentially dangerous equipment (pilots and nuclear plant engineers). They have also permitted direct-observation urine sampling, even when the observer was of the other sex and even when less intrusive methods of sampling exist.[3]

The video monitors, the random checks, and the general atmosphere of suspicion fostered by the measures taken at Saint Catherine's do not produce a positive working environment. In fact, they may contribute to just the behavior employers want to curb, on the grounds that if workers constantly feel mistrusted, they may come to feel under less obligation to warrant an employer's trust. Yet intrusive monitoring of employees is becoming much more widespread. It is common for supervisors to listen to telephone marketing calls, for example "to assure quality," but also to pressure employees to work more productively and avoid personal communication on company time. It is also increasingly common for employers to have access to the computer files, e-mail, and voice mail communications of their staff and sometimes to monitor these. It has been reported that 30 percent of three hundred companies surveyed routinely search their employees' files and communications (Pillar, 1993).

---

[3] See, for example, *Wilcher v. City of Wilmington*, in which a group of firefighters argued unsuccessfully that the city had no right to force them to urinate in front of a stranger for purposes of random drug testing. The court found for the city on the ground that the observer was necessary to ensure that the test was reliable.

The companies argue that this monitoring promotes productivity while enabling them to detect and punish abuses. But employees like Angie see this as humiliating, and many find it generates severe psychological stresses and even physical symptoms.

Related ethical problems involve what, exactly, an employer or potential employer is entitled to know about employees. Consider this case.

Case 10.5: Confidentiality Between Present and Potential Employer

According to medical center policy, Carol H. has recently been disciplined for a series of medication administration errors. Although she is not in danger of losing her job, she is quite uncomfortable with her nurse manager, who, Carol feels, dislikes and distrusts her. So Carol has applied for employment at a nearby medical center because she wants to practice with a "clean slate." However, on her application, she is required to list her current supervisor.

The nurse manager of Carol's prospective unit contacts Carol's current supervisor to get the "scoop" on Carol before Carol is actually hired. In the course of the conversation, Carol's supervisor casually informs the prospective nurse manager of Carol's recent discipline. Is this a breach of confidentiality?

For hiring purposes, employers are generally prohibited from inquiring into matters that have historically led to discrimination, such as religious preference, race, or age. However, it is likely that Carol's application may be turned down once her prospective employer learns of the recent medication errors. Should her recent problems be considered relevant and appropriate information for a prospective employer to know? Protecting patients from unprofessional practice is certainly very important. But Carol's current employer is not prepared to fire Carol for these medication errors, only to discipline her. That implies that Carol's employer does not consider these errors serious enough to place patients at significant risk. Carol wants to move on because of tensions between herself and her supervisor, not because her practice is considered seriously dangerous. Should future employers be "scared off" by a supervisor's casual remarks—remarks that may represent dislike or distrust as much as or more than an objective professional appraisal of Carol's practice?

Once more, the goal of limiting access to certain information about prospective employees is to reduce the likelihood of unjust discrimination in hiring. And, in fact, it may turn out that Carol would have a legal grievance against her supervisor for this breach of confidentiality, though the issue is not at all clear. Yet current hiring procedures routinely generate a huge repertoire of factors that can be and often are used to discriminate against some prospective employees. For example, employers often require applicants to fill out exhaustive questionnaires on medical status, health history, and the like; and the results of these inquiries are widely used to guide hiring decisions. An increasing number of employers will not hire smokers. And while health histories have primarily been used to make sure that a prospective employee was not disqualified from performing effectively because of some relevant health problem, they are now increasingly being used to screen out those potential employees most likely to make use of expensive health or other benefits or whose genetic makeup or health history might place them at risk of job-related injury and place their companies at greater legal liability. Even more intrusive, as well as even less predictably valid, are the batteries of personality inventories, honesty and loyalty tests, and related psychological measurements of "institutional fit" for employment.

We believe that policies concerning workplace information, drug, health, and other testing should be guided by the same ethical decision-making perspectives that we have advocated throughout this book. That is, we think that respect for the autonomy of employees should not be ignored in favor of the interests of employers, though employer and patient interests are obviously also important. Since practical limitations prevent many health care workers from freely shopping for an employer whose values match their own, most testing occurs in a highly coercive environment without truly informed consent (especially, as with e-mail monitoring, when employees are unaware of the intrusions). It is also probable that those who are most likely to need employment and are least able to move if dissatisfied are also those most likely to be subject to testing (nursing assistants, for example, or environmental services staff are far more likely to be screened than is the hospital legal counsel or an orthopedic surgeon). So it is important to protect employees from irresponsible intrusions and to protect their privacy, just as it is important to protect the confidentiality of patients.

What is needed is a policy that responsibly protects the most important interests of all parties insofar as that is possible. Genuine consultation with all affected parties in developing such policies is, once more, a fruitful approach. As a practical matter, testing needs to be job-related, and it needs to address a genuine need or problem in an effective way. It needs to be done with sympathetic understanding that not all previous job tensions need to reflect badly on applicants, though it needs to take seriously those problems that may affect job performance. It needs to be done with as much respect for privacy as possible; for example, there are ways to assure the reliability of a urine sample without directly observing the person producing the sample. And extreme care needs to be exerted to avoid introducing new forms of unjust discrimination by means of employee testing. The cure for increased workplace risk is a safer workplace for all, not creation of a caste of pariahs whose genetic makeup makes them unemployable.

QUESTIONS FOR DISCUSSION

1. Suppose that you are responsible for developing policies to address the problems at Saint Catherine's. How would you go about doing that? Specifically, what would you recommend?

2. Some companies currently require applicants to submit samples of their hair for analysis. Such samples can reveal traces of drugs over a 90-day period, as opposed to the 2–3 days typically derived from urine samples. Hair can also be used to test genetic makeup in order to identify some potential disease problems. Is this an ethically responsible job requirement?

3. More generally, what do you think your employer has an ethical entitlement to know about you? Do you think each of the following is "fair game"? If so, explain why; if not, explain why not. (a) Age? (b) Past performance appraisals from previous employers? (c) Academic credentials? (d) Grades (and withdrawals) from all your courses? (e) Marital status? (f) Credit history? (g) Criminal record? (h) Driving history? (i) Disabilities? (j) Comprehensive health history? (k) Comprehensive genetic screening? (l) Whether you have ever stolen anything? (m) Whether you might lie about having stolen something?

CONFIDENTIALITY AND QUALITY OF CARE

There are also ethically troubling confidentiality cases that arise among health care workers concerning quality of care. Hospitals routinely monitor surgical cases to assure successful outcomes, and they also monitor billing and other matters. But so do such agencies as the Joint Commission for Accrediting Health Organizations (JCAHO). In fact, JCAHO requires that events posing serious safety threats to patients be reported to the agency as part of the "quality improvement process." Hospitals that fail to report are subject to citation and, ultimately, to revocation of their accreditation, with dire financial consequences. However, each health care facility itself is responsible for determining whether a particular event is considered a *sentinel event*, which is a problem that actually has to be reported. Further, because health care facilities are encouraged to correct problems that lead to errors and mishaps themselves, the investigation of problem cases is considered confidential unless they are reported to JCAHO or a grievance resolution forum, such as an institutional ethics committee, or, in the worst case, to an attorney. Now, consider this case.

Case 10.6: Confidentiality and Credentialing Agency Expectations

Manfred Zerkin has bilateral degenerative joint disease of both hips and is scheduled to have total joint replacement surgery. The side with the least disease is the side the surgeon recommends be done first. Mr. Zerkin agrees to the surgery and is scheduled for a right hip arthroplasty. On the day of the surgery, Mr. Zerkin signs the permission for the surgeon to perform a *left* hip arthroplasty. When the nurse asks him what he is having done, he informs her that he is "having my hip fixed." In a nutshell, Mr. Zerkin has surgery on the wrong hip first.

Is Mr. Zerkin's case a sentinel event that would need to be reported? Almost certainly, the hospital risk manager will argue that since he was going to have both hips repaired anyway, Zerkin's situation should not be considered a wrong-site surgery. Instead, it should be categorized as a "near miss" that does not need to be reported. All parties to the event are likely to be instructed to keep the details in confidence, treating the matter as an internal quality-improvement activity. Treating the problem this way has another benefit from the risk manager's perspective. As long as the incident is not disclosed, it is protected from discovery under the law. This means that a zealous attorney or greedy family member is much less likely to be able to sue the hospital and the surgeon for malpractice.

> A sentinel event *is one that represents a bona fide quality-of-care breach that brought harm to a patient. An example is amputation of the wrong limb or wrongful death due to a medication error. Sentinel events must be reported. The result of reporting sentinel events can be a survey by one of the credentialing agencies. And if the survey uncovers problems in care delivery, it is possible that the health care facility would lose its Medicare/ Medicaid reimbursement status. Loss of this status really means closure of the facility because most third-party payers will follow reimbursement decisions of Medicare and Medicaid.*

Nevertheless, an ethical problem arises: Should this event be disclosed and, if so, to whom? We think the patient and his family have an ethical claim to this information. To conceal it or deny it violates Mr. Zerkin's autonomy. Even though such disclosure may put the hospital at some risk for a lawsuit, it also offers the opportunity for a cooperative or mediated resolution. Besides, not disclosing leaves the door just as open for the dreaded lawsuit while escalating the hospital's appearance of guilt. But JCAHO places hospitals in an awkward position regarding cases like Mr. Zerkin's. If the matter does not come to JCAHO's attention, a tremendous amount of time and energy will be saved. But if it does, accrediting officials will sift through this and related cases and impose correction plans that may be expensive, onerous, and time-consuming. That process does not create much incentive to report events that might be passed off as near misses rather than sentinel events.

Problems regarding disclosing practice or other professional issues within or outside of health care agencies abound. Consider this case.

Case 10.7: Whistle-Blowing on Creative Billing

Barry A. is a home-health aide who has been working for Midwest Homecare for about nine months. Midwest is not doing well financially, and Barry's supervisor, Ruth M., has encouraged Barry and the home-care staff to think "creatively" about how to document their services, bearing in mind that the financial health of Midwest is the only job security they have. Because reimbursement levels from Medicare are so low and so many services are disallowed, Ruth, who is under heavy pressure from finance, regularly "upcodes" and "unbundles" services to secure reimbursements that meet Midwest's costs. Barry is uncomfortable with this, but he needs his job. What should he do?

According to the U.S. Department of Justice, fraud accounts for as much as 10 percent of the nation's health care expenses. Moreover, the Government Accounting Office (GAO), which looked at 80 randomly selected home-health benefit claims from California, found that 46 of them should have been partially or totally denied, an example the GAO takes to be representative of the industry (Polston, 1999). While many instances of fraud certainly are motivated by greed, many are not; some fraud is committed because it seems to be the only way to meet the needs of patients—at least in the eyes of the perpetrators. When Medicare reimburses below costs, health care organizations may feel justified in manipulating the system for more equitable reimbursement levels.

Three ways of doing this seem especially common. *Upcoding* is filing a claim with the Health Care Financing Administration that describes services reimbursed at higher rates than are the services actually performed. So Ruth might upcode Brian's 30-minute home-care visit to a 50-minute visit because the reimbursement for the longer visit might actually meet Midwest's costs. *Unbundling* is filing a separate claim for individual services that are usually performed and billed together. The reason to unbundle is that individual services are often reimbursed at a higher level than when they are billed as part of a single, comprehensive service. Falsifying cost reports occurs when providers try to get paid for unallowable costs by describing them as procedures that can be reimbursed. An example might be filing marketing expenses as patient education.

> *It is common practice to bill for surgical procedures by time, usually in 15-minute increments. Thus, if a surgery lasts 30 minutes or less, it is usually billed for 30 minutes even when it may have taken only 15 minutes. Is this an ethical issue?*

> *Health care facilities often offer community education about disease or therapies. Suppose that Elsewhere Medical Center offers a luncheon program to community members in order to introduce a new procedure to a patient population who will benefit from this procedure. Is this education, marketing, or a bit of both?*

Now, what should Brian do? He may have considerable sympathy with the motives that cause Ruth to falsify her billing. But fraud is more than a little dishonest; it's unlawful. Not only is he running a risk of legal liability by going along with it, but he also does not want to work for an agency that engages in this kind of behavior. He strongly suspects that talking about his concerns with Ruth would be unproductive, would mark him as not being a "team player," and might lead to his termination. Besides he needs this job; he just doesn't want to have to break the law to keep it.

He has a number of options. Midwest, or Midwest's parent corporation, almost certainly has a corporate compliance hot line. Brian could call that hot line, report the situation anonymously, and the situation would be investigated by Ruth's supervisor or someone else in an appropriate position. But Ruth will probably find out about Brian's call, and she may retaliate. If Brian were to be fired or otherwise disciplined for his actions, he would have recourse through the National Labor Relations Board, which would almost certainly order his reinstatement with at least his back pay and interest. Still, going through such an experience is a high price to pay for professionalism.

Another approach, under the Federal False Claims Act, would be to file a lawsuit under seal with a court. As long as the suit is under seal,

Midwest will not find out. Brian would then have to provide documentation of all the information he has about the fraud he thinks is going on, and the government would have 60 days to investigate and decide whether to prosecute. Since 1986, whistle-blowers have been entitled to receive a 15–25 percent portion of what the government recovers. But once again, such a filing imposes a heavy personal cost. And some job and antiretaliation protections apply only when the fraud exposed is committed against the federal government. Most states still do not have adequate protections for health care professionals who blow the whistle.

Once more, what should Brian do? Brian's case involves serious legal questions, and we do not presume to advise him on those. Instead, we recommend that he take them to the agency's legal counsel for advice and also contact the state nursing association regarding the legal situation. Meanwhile, we recommend working within the system—inside Midwest and its parent corporation—so far as possible and until it actually is futile. As health care agencies become more legally cautious, they are also becoming more aware that ethical concerns can affect or even create legal liabilities, which amount to powerful incentives to settle problems cooperatively rather than in an adversarial proceeding.

QUESTIONS FOR DISCUSSION

1. What would you do in Mr. Zerkin's case? Give a persuasive ethical justification for your resolution of the problem.

2. What would you do in Brian's case? Give a persuasive ethical justification for your resolution of the problem.

3. Why is whistle-blowing so costly to the whistle-blower? What are some responsible ways to resolve concerns about unethical or unlawful practices short of "going public"? Do you think health care staff ought to be financially rewarded for blowing the whistle on their employers? Why or why not?

REFERENCES

American Nurses' Association. 1985/1994. The code for nurses with interpretive statements. In *Association of operating room nurses: Standards, recommended practices, and guidelines* (1999). Denver, Colo.: AORN.

Bayley, S. C., and Cranford, R. E. 1986. Ethics committees: What we have learned. In *Making choices: Ethical issues for health care professionals*, edited by E. Friedman. Chicago: American Hospital Publishing.

Beauchamps, D. E. 1986. Public health as social justice. In *Biomedical ethics*, 2d ed., edited by T. A. Mappes and J. S. Zembaty. New York: McGraw-Hill.

Benjamin, M., and Curtis, J. 1992. *Ethics in nursing*, 3d ed. New York: Oxford University Press.

Bentham, J. 1789-1948. *Introduction to the principles of morals and legislation*, edited by W. Harrison. Oxford: Oxford University Press.

Bloom, M. 1998. Physician's income climbs again. *Physicians Weekly* 15(12).

Brandt, R. 1981. W. K. Frankena and ethics of virtue. *The Monist*.

Brook, R., et al. 1990. Predicting the appropriate use of carotid endarterectomy, upper gastrointestinal endoscopy, and coronary angioplasty. *New England Journal of Medicine* 323(17).

Deloughery, G. 1991. *Issues and trends in nursing*. St. Louis: Mosby.

Dubos, R. 1961. *Mirage of health*. Garden City, N.Y.: Doubleday.

English, J. 1975. Abortion and the concept of person. *The Canadian Journal of Philosophy* 5(2).

Feinberg, J. 1965. Psychological egoism. In *Reason and responsibility*, edited by J. Feinberg. Encino, Calif.: Dickenson.

Frankena, W. 1973. *Ethics*, 2d ed. Englewood Cliffs N.J.: Prentice-Hall.

Gilligan, C. 1982. *In a different voice*. Cambridge: Harvard University Press.

Joint Commission on Accreditation of Health Care Organizations. 1998. *1998 hospital accreditation standards*. Oakbrook Terrace, Ill.: JCAHO.

Kitchner, P. 1996. *The lives to come*. New York: Simon and Schuster.

Lessenberry, J. 1996. Dr. K[evorkian] ignoring his professed assisted-suicide guidelines. *Oakland Press*, October 20.

Lowe, S. 1996. "Cleaning up" after Kevorkian. *South Bend Tribune*, October 16.

Lynn, J. 1984. Roles and functions of institutional ethics committees. In *Institutional ethics committees and health care decision making*, edited by R. E. Cranford and A. E. Doudera. Ann Arbor, Mich.: Health Administration Press.

MacIntyre, A. 1984. *After virtue*. South Bend, Ind.: Notre Dame University Press.

———. 1966. *A short history of ethics*. New York: Collier Books.

———. 1989. *Whose justice? Which rationality?* South Bend, Ind.: Notre Dame University Press.

McAuley, C. Circa 1831. Mercy values. Farmington Hills, Mich.: Mercy Health Services.

Medlin, B. 1957. Ultimate principles and ethical egoism. *Australasian Journal of Philosophy* 35.

The Merck manual of diagnosis and therapy, 16th ed., edited by R. Berkow. 1992. Rahway, N.J.: Merck, Sharpe, and Dohme Research Laboratories.

Mullett, S. 1989. Shifting perspectives: A new approach to ethics. In *Feminist perspectives*, edited by L. Code, S. Mullett, and C. Overal. Toronto: University of Toronto.

Nightingale, F. 1859/1993. *Notes on nursing*. Philadelphia: Lippincott.

Noddings, N. 1984. *Caring: A feminine approach to ethics and moral education*. Berkeley: University of California Press.

Nyberg, D. 1993. *The varnished truth*. Chicago: University of Chicago Press.

Oliner, S. P., and Oliner, P. M. 1988. *The altruistic personality*. New York: Viking Press.

People's Medical Society. 1996. Keep it confidential. *People's Medical Society News Letter* 15(3).

Pence, G. E. 1990. *Classic cases in medical ethics*. New York: McGraw-Hill.

Pillar, C. 1993. Bosses with x-ray eyes. *Macworld*, July.

Polston, M. D. 1999. Whistleblowing: Does the law protect you? *American Journal of Nursing* 99(1): 26–32.

President's Commission. (1984). Decision to forgo life-sustaining treatment. Washington, D.C.: Author.

Ross, W. 1939. *The right and the good*. Oxford: Clarendon Press.

Sagan, S. 1989. *The limits of morality*. Oxford: Clarendon Press.

Singer, P. 1975. *Animal liberation: A new ethics for our treatment of animals*. New York: Avon.

———. 1979. *Practical ethics*. Cambridge: Cambridge University Press.

Southwick, A. F. 1979. *The law of hospital and health care administration*. Ann Arbor, Mich.: Health Administration Press.

Stark, F. H. 1993. Protective safer medical devices. *Congressional Record*, h1077–78, March 9.

Steinbock, B., and McClamrock, R. 1994. When is birth unfair to the child? *Hastings Center Report* 24(6): 15–21.

Temkin, O., and Temkin, C. L. 1967. *Ancient medicine: Selected papers of Ludwig Edelstein*. Baltimore: Johns Hopkins University Press.

Tong, R. 1997. *Feminist approaches to bioethics*. Boulder, Colo.: Westview Press.

Veatch, R. 1974. Who should pay for smokers' medical care? *Hastings Center Report* 4: 8–9.

Wall, S. D., Olcott, E. W., and Gerberding, J. L. 1991. AIDS risk and risk reduction in the radiology department. *American Journal of Roentgenology* 157: 911–17.

Washington et al. v. Harold Glucksberg, 117 S. Ct. 2258.

INDEX

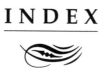